THERAPEUTIC
NUTRITION

THERAPEUTIC NUTRITION

A practical guide

DR C. R. PENNINGTON

King's Cross Hospital
Dundee
Scotland

SPRINGER-SCIENCE+
BUSINESS MEDIA, B.V.

© C. R. Pennington 1988
Originally published by Chapman and Hall in 1988

ISBN 978-0-412-29230-9   ISBN 978-1-4899-7108-1 (eBook)
DOI 10.1007/978-1-4899-7108-1

British Library Cataloguing in Publication Data

Pennington, C. R.
    Therapeutic nutrition : a practical guide.
    1. Diet therapy   2. Nutrition
    I. Title
    615.8'54   RM216

CONTENTS

PREFACE

Although the subject of nutrition is of major importance in most branches of medicine it has only recently attracted the attention of many clinicians and still receives little emphasis in the undergraduate curricula of most medical schools. There is now an increasing appreciation of the role of nutrition in the pathogenesis of many forms of chronic disease and the development of methods of nutritional support for the management of intestinal failure represents one of the most important and least heralded advances in therapeutics. This book is intended as a source of practical information on therapeutic nutrition. I hope it will be of value to the senior undergraduate who is learning about clinical practice, and the junior doctor who is training for postgraduate diplomas.

I wish to express my thanks to my secretary, Miss Alison McIntosh, for her invaluable help in deciphering and typing the manuscript, to Miss Maureen Sneddon of the Department of Medical Illustration, Ninewells Hospital, for help with the illustrations and to my wife, Jane, for her support and professional dietetic advice.

1

INTRODUCTION

The subject of nutrition is relevant to the entire spectrum of medical practice. Under-nutrition, over-nutrition and inappropriate nutrition are all major factors in the pathogenesis of disease. Disease frequently leads to malnutrition. In hospital practice nutritional therapy is primarily concerned with the treatment of malnutrition and with the prevention and management of disease.

Following the discovery of vitamins, the description of vitamin deficiency syndromes and the recognition of the features of protein energy malnutrition, the subject of nutrition attracted little further medical interest and has been given little emphasis in the under graduate medical curriculum. Consequently medical graduates frequently have no concept of the importance of nutrition and poor understanding of dietetics. Nevertheless the same people are given responsibility for the supervision of ill and post-operative patients. It is not surprising that under-nutrition escapes recognition until malnutrition is severe. Many studies have shown that malnutrition is common in hospital practice, in both medical and surgical patients in Britain and the USA. Frequently nutritional status deteriorates during in-patient management: this applies particularly to surgical practice. Consequently many patients are at increased risk of complications such as infection and delayed wound healing which in turn impose additional nutritional demands. Common errors of nutritional management include a delay in establishing nutritional support, the failure to utilize fully the enteral route, and inexpert administration of parenteral nutrition which is expensive in terms of cost, resources and morbidity.

The recent resurgence of interest in the problem of malnutrition in hospital practice is attributable to a variety of factors. These include the recognition that malnutrition is common in hospital patients and the realization that weight loss is associated with morbidity and mortality in addition to that attributable to underlying disease. The emergence of gastroenterology as a speciality and the increased incidence of intestinal disease such as Crohn's disease has led to the concept of intestinal failure. This in turn has stimulated the development of methods of nutritional support. Finally the introduction of more aggressive forms of surgical and medical treatment and the development of intensive care have increased the number of patients with multi-system failure who require nutritional therapy as part of their management.

Nutritional advisory groups and nutritional support teams have been formed in many hospitals by interested members of staff to develop and apply nutritional support techniques. The composition of a nutritional support team is outlined in Table 1.1. The members have individual and collective responsibilities. The anaesthetist supervises the nutritional management of patients in the intensive care unit and is frequently called upon to insert temporary central venous catheters. The biochemist is responsible for biochemical monitoring which is particularly important in patients who require prolonged total parenteral nutrition and those with severe malnutrition or organ failure. The dietitian is involved in patient monitoring and advising on the provision of macro- and micronutrients particularly in patients with anorexia, malabsorption and those who are being transferred from parenteral to enteral feeding. In addition, the dietitian is normally responsible for the selection of enteral feeds. The nurse supervises catheter care techniques and the administration of naso-enteral feeding. The pharmacist advises on nutrient compatibility and is responsible for the compounding of parenteral solutions. Occasional recourse to the microbiologist is also required during episodes of catheter-related sepsis.

The collective responsibilities of the nutrition team are outlined in Table 1.2. A dynamic team can be very effective in a variety of ways. Increasingly one of the most pressing responsibilities is cost containment. This is facilitated by limiting the range of enteral feeds to be stocked by the pharmacy and encouraging the use of the less expensive polymeric preparations where possible. Economies are also achieved by the careful selection of patients for parenteral nutrition and

Table 1.1 The composition of the nutritional support team

Anaesthetist
Biochemist
Clinician
Dietitian
Nurse
Pharmacist

Table 1.2 Some areas of responsibility of the nutritional support team

Patient monitoring
Selection of enteral feeds
Patient selection for parenteral nutrition
The provision of parenteral nutrients
The development and implementation of catheter care protocols

employing a limited range of standard compounded bags which will meet the nutritional needs of most of these patients. Of more importance is the reduction in complications and patient morbidity associated with nutritional support. The introduction of careful catheter care protocols will virtually eliminate catheter-related sepsis, previously a major and common problem during parenteral nutrition. This achieves a significant indirect cost saving. Finally the group should serve an important role in the education and in-service training of nursing and medical staff who are thus kept informed of the rapid advances in techniques of nutritional support.

Major developments have occurred in the methods of nutritional support and in the management of intestinal failure. A wide range of enteral feeds, including polymeric, peptide and elemental diets, is now commercially available and can be delivered through modern safe fine bore naso-gastric tubes. These are well tolerated and unlike earlier wide bore tubes they do not cause oesophageal damage. The use of home nocturnal naso-enteral hyperalimentation, in which patients are taught to pass nasogastric tubes each night and infuse nutrient solutions while they sleep, has greatly increased intestinal availability and reduced the need for parenteral feeding in patients with borderline intestinal function. The administration of parenteral nutrition has been simplified and made safer by the introduction of compounded nutrient solutions in collapsible plastic bags and improvements in catheter design. Following the introduction of careful catheter care protocols the problem of catheter infection has been virtually overcome and patients who require long-term parenteral nutrition can safely be managed at home.

There is now general acceptance that many of the degenerative diseases which afflict Western societies and which remain uncommon or rare in countries of the Third World may be related to diet. Examples include obesity, cardiovascular disease, diverticular disease and intestinal cancer. Attention has been focused on the need to improve the national diet. On the basis of current knowledge broadly similar nutritional guidelines have been issued by the Word Health Organization, the UK Department of Health and Social Security, and the National Advisory Committee on Nutritional Education. A significant reduction in the consumption of fat, especially saturated fat, is recommended. There should be an increase in the proportion of energy obtained from carbohydrate with the consumption of more unrefined carbohydrate and thus fibre, and a reduction in the intake of sugar. The need for such improvements in nutritional standards has received scant attention by many clinicians. This represents a lost opportunity for health education which might be expected to exert a beneficial influence on future disease trends.

There has been a resurgence of interest in the dietary management of many diseases. These include renal failure, hyperlipidaemia, and Crohn's disease, as well as gluten enteropathy and inborn errors of metabolism. There is also widespread popular interest but little scientific data about food intolerance which remains a grey area of definition, diagnosis and management.

This book is written as a practical guide for medical undergraduates and newly qualified doctors, and it will also be of interest to dietitians and nurses who are involved in hospital practice. It is primarily concerned with the recognition, significance and management of malnutrition in hospital practice, and the importance of nutrition in the prevention and management of disease. The following two chapters describe basic nutritional physiology and biochemistry, food nutrients and dietary requirements. Three chapters are then devoted to clinical malnutrition and the principles of enteral and parenteral nutrition. The next chapter discusses nutrition in specific disease, and this is followed by a chapter on dietetic management. The final chapter discusses the expanding subject of drugs and nutrition. The book is not intended as a textbook of dietetics, and paediatric nutrition has not been covered. No attempt has been made to discuss the pressing and as yet insoluble problem of malnutrition in the Third World. Such a subject is beyond the scope of this text.

2

PHYSIOLOGY AND BIOCHEMISTRY IN THE NORMAL AND MALNOURISHED

The human body is a complex compartmentalized structure whose major constituents participate in a continuous metabolic flux. Normal function, health and survival depend upon the adequate provision of essential nutrients to fuel metabolic functions and maintain structural integrity. Large nutrient reserves are normally available and during starvation may be conserved by processes of adaption. Adaptive mechanisms are disrupted during stress such as burns, trauma or sepsis when accelerated nutritional depletion may jeopardize the patient's recovery. An understanding of the basic principles of body composition and metabolic biochemistry is important for the successful nutritional management of patients.

2.1 Body composition

The gross composition of a 70 kg male is shown in Table 2.1.

There is a wide variation in composition between different subjects, particularly with reference to fat stores. Body composition is influenced significantly by sex and age. Female subjects possess considerably more fat, and correspondingly less water. A gradual

Table 2.1 The gross composition of a 70 kg male

Substance	Weight (kg)	% of total body weight
Water	43	62
Protein	12	17
Fat	10	14
Minerals	4	6
Carbohydrates	1	1
Vitamins	Trace amounts	

(Modified from Davidson and Passmore (1986): *Human Nutrition and Dietetics*)

reduction in muscle bulk occurs after 40 years of age, and calcium content may also be reduced, particularly in elderly females. However an increase in fat stores usually means that body weight remains constant or increases with age.

2.1.1 BODY WATER

A relative increase in the proportion of body water occurs in malnutrition. Inevitable water loss occurs through the skin and respiratory tract. Whereas these losses usually amount to one litre a day they vary considerably according to prevailing conditions and much greater losses happen in pyrexial, burnt and tachypnoeic patients. A further 0.5 litre is the minimal requirement to excrete waste products in the urine, but greater urinary losses occur in hypermetabolic patients and those with renal impairment.

Losses of up to 10% of the body water can occur. Significant losses are usually accompanied by an equivalent depletion of electrolytes and lead to impaired organ function, particularly renal failure.

2.1.2 PROTEIN

Almost 50% of body protein is found in muscle and 25% in supporting structures such as the skin and skeleton. Other proteins function as enzymes, and in the blood proteins fulfil important roles in transport, immune defence and the maintenance of osmotic gradients.

Proteins are composed of chains of amino acids the sequence of which determines their three-dimensional structure. There are 20 amino acids, nine of which cannot be adequately synthesized and must be supplied. These are known as the essential amino acids. They are discussed further in Chapter 3.

Muscle protein provides an energy reserve for gluconeogenesis. This occurs particularly in stressed patients, and in the absence of adequate nutritional support their illness may be accompanied by severe muscle wasting.

2.1.3 FAT

Lipids are water insoluble substances which include triglycerides, phospholipids and sterols. The vast majority of lipid is in the form of triglyceride in adipose tissue the main function of which is as an energy store.

(a) Triglycerides

Triglycerides are esters of glycerol with fatty acids, and their basic structure is shown in Fig. 2.1.

$$CH_2-O-CO-R_1$$
$$CH-O-CO-R_2$$
$$CH_2-O-CO-R_3$$

Figure 2.1 The basic formula for triglycerides

Fatty acids are classified in three groups. Some are saturated without double bonds, some are mono-unsaturated with one double bond, others are polyunsaturated. Some examples of these fatty acids are shown in Table 2.2. The polyunsaturated fatty acids linoleic,

Table 2.2 Examples of fatty acids

Type	Fatty acid
Saturated	Palmitic, stearic
Mono-unsaturated	Oleic
Polyunsaturated	Linoleic, linolenic

linolenic, and arachidonic acids are considered essential as they cannot be synthesized, although arachidonic acid can be formed from linoleic acid.

(b) Phospholipids

Phospholipids such as lecithin and sphingomyelin have an important role in cell membranes.

(c) Sterols

Sterols include cholesterol and sex hormones. Bile acids are synthesized from cholesterol.

2.1.4 MINERALS

The mineral content may conveniently be considered in three groups. The body contains more than 100 mg of the major minerals, up to 20 mg of the minor minerals, and very small amounts of the trace elements. Examples of the body minerals are listed in Table 2.3.

Calcium accounts for 45% of the total mineral content and phosphorus for 25%. The majority of these elements are found in the skeleton. Most of the iodine is present in the thyroid gland and a majority of iron is incorporated into haemoglobin.

Many of these elements have important metabolic functions which will be considered in Section 2.4.5. Their requirements will be considered in more detail in Chapter 3.

Table 2.3 The body content of some elements

Group 1 (>100 mg)	Group 2 (1–20 mg)	Group 3 (<1 mg)
Calcium	Magnesium	Copper
Phosphorus	Silicon	Manganese
Sulphur	Iron	Iodide
Potassium	Zinc	Chromium
Sodium	Fluoride	Cobalt
Chloride		Selenium

2.1.5 CARBOHYDRATES

Most of the carbohydrate is found in the polysaccharide storage form glycogen in the liver and muscles. There is approximately 100 g of glycogen in the liver and 300 g in muscles. Carbohydrates are also important components of complex molecules such as deoxyribonucleic acid and ribonucleic acid. Small amounts exist in the form of monosaccharides, particularly glucose.

2.1.6 VITAMINS

Vitamins play an important role in metabolic processes. They are essential coenzymes in connective tissue, haematinic, purine and protein energy metabolism, and are present in trace amounts. The liver is an important storage organ for Vitamin A, Vitamin B12 and folate. Vitamin D and Vitamin E are stored in the fat depots. The vitamin status of an average male is illustrated in Table 2.4.

Table 2.4 The body pool of selected vitamins in an average male

Vitamin	Body pool (mg)
Vitamin C	2500
Vitamin A	400
Vitamin B6	25
Folate	25
Vitamin B12	3

(Adapted from Kelleher, J. (1984) The composition of the body, *Hospital Up-Date*, **10**, 729–34)

2.2 Body compartments

The body can be divided into three compartments: the cell mass, extracellular supporting tissue, and fat reserves. The extracellular supporting tissue consists of: blood plasma, interstitial fluid, supporting tissues and the skeleton.

The relative size of these compartments varies in health and disease. They are not defined by static boundaries but are in a state of dynamic equilibrium with constant metabolic exchange and tissue renewal. The body compartments are summarized in Fig. 2.2.

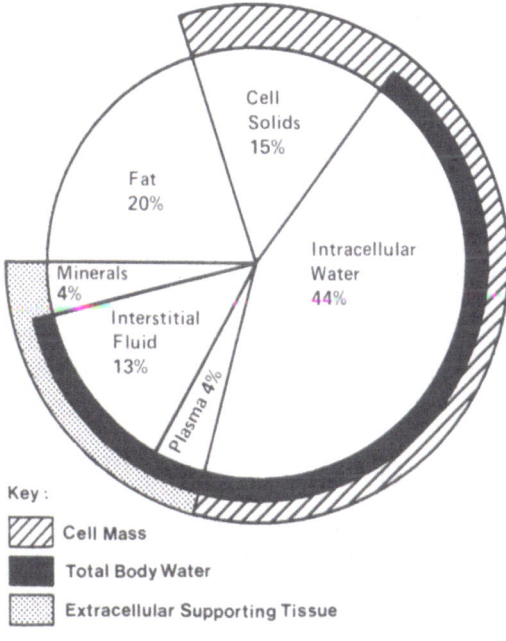

Figure 2.2 A summary of body compartments

Table 2.5 Electrolyte content of extracellular and intracellular fluid (values expressed in mmol/1)

	Extracellular fluid	Intracellular fluid
Cations		
Na	145	10
K	4.5	150
Ca	2	2
Mg	1	7
Anions		
Cl	100	10
HCO$_3$	25	10
PO$_4$	1	40
SO$_4$	0.2	5

Important differences exist in electrolyte distribution between the intracellular fluid and the extracellular fluid which is composed of the interstitial fluid and plasma. The chemical composition of these compartments is summarized in Table 2.5.

2.3 Fuel composition

The body can utilize three major sources of fuel to provide energy which is stored in the form of adenosine triphosphate (ATP) and is used for the maintenance of structure and function. These sources are glucose, fatty acids and amino acids. They are respectively derived from glycogen, fat and protein which may be regarded as fuel stores.

2.3.1 GLYCOGEN

Glycogen stores are very small (as discussed in Section 2.1.5). Hepatic glycogen is sufficient to maintain blood glucose for only very short periods without replenishment. Muscle glycogen cannot be converted to blood glucose because muscle tissue lacks the enzyme glucose-6 phosphatase, and is conserved to meet the energy demands of vigorous exercise and anoxia. Furthermore for each gram of glycogen 1-2 g of intracellular water accumulates with associated electrolytes. Therefore on a weight basis glycogen only provides 25–30% of its theoretical 4 kcal/g. Consequently it is not an efficient storage medium.

2.3.2 PROTEIN

Protein serves structural, contractile and enzymatic functions, hence there is a need to conserve protein stores. Like glycogen, protein is in an aqueous phase and tissue contains 25% protein by weight. Thus protein is also inefficient as an energy source on a unit weight basis.

2.3.3 FAT

Fat is the main energy and source provides 9 kcal/g. The other functions of insulation and protection are of limited importance.

Whereas energy may be derived from all three sources, some tissues require glucose notably the nervous system, the haemopoietic system and the renal medulla. During periods of prolonged starvation metabolic adaption ensures the preferential utilization of fat and the conservation of valuable protein stores. These adaptive mechanisms break down in stress associated with infection, surgery or trauma, leading to protein depletion and severe muscle wasting.

2.4 Metabolic biochemistry

The physiological functions including protein synthesis, secretion, the maintenance of electrochemical gradients and locomotion all require energy. This is stored in chemical form as adenosine triphosphate (ATP).

ATP is produced from adenosine diphosphate and inorganic phosphate as the result of the oxidation of glucose, fatty acids and ketones. Some tissues such as liver and skeletal muscle are able to metabolize fat, but others, including the central nervous system and haemopoietic system, require glucose.

2.4.1 THE TRICARBOXYLIC ACID CYCLE

The catabolism of glucose and fatty acids provides a limited amount of ATP. Most ATP is generated through the tricarboxylic acid cycle which occurs in the mitochondria. The tricarboxylic acid cycle is entered by derivatives of glucose and amino acid metabolism and it produces reduced intermediates such as $NADH_2$ and $FADH_2$. The subsequent oxidation of these reduced equivalents is linked to the formation of ATP by oxidative phosphorylation.

The tricarboxylic acid cycle is summarized in Fig. 2.3. It serves two functions:

- The generation of ATP
- The formation of precursors for synthetic pathways

For example oxaloacetate and alpha ketoglutarate are precursors for the amino acids aspartate and glutamate.

2.4.2 CARBOHYDRATE METABOLISM

Glucose may be metabolized in three pathways:

- Oxidation to glucuronic acid which after phosphorylation enters the 'alternative pathway' (see below)
- Reduction to sorbitol which is subsequently oxidized to fructose

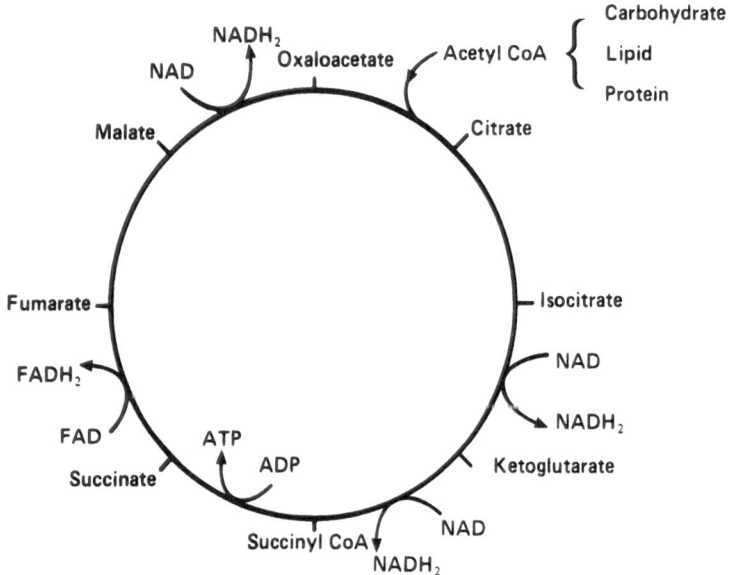

Figure 2.3 Summary of the tricarboxylic acid cycle

- The majority is metabolized through the 'major pathway' to glucose-6 phosphate. Most of the galactose and fructose are metabolized through glucose-6 phosphate.

Glucose-6 phosphate may be metabolized in four ways:

- Hydrolysis to glucose and phosphate: this occurs in the liver, kidney and intestine
- Conversion to glucose-1 phosphate for the synthesis of poly-saccharides such as glycogen: this process needs energy and occurs in the liver and muscle
- Oxidation to 6-phosphogluconic acid: this is the start of the 'alternative pathway'
- Isomerization to fructose-6-phosphate: this is the main pathway of glucose oxidation via glycolysis and the tricarboxylic acid cycle

(a) Glycolysis

This process, the Embden-Meyerhof pathway, occurs in the cyto-plasm and involves many intermediates through which glucose and other carbohydrates are metabolized to pyruvate. Under aerobic conditions pyruvate enters the mitochondria where it is converted to acetyl CoA through which it enters the tricarboxylic acid cycle, it is converted to lactate under hypoxic conditions. This pathway is shown diagrammatically in Fig. 2.4.

This process provides a limited amount of ATP. Although the formation of lactate reduces the net ATP supply it serves to provide

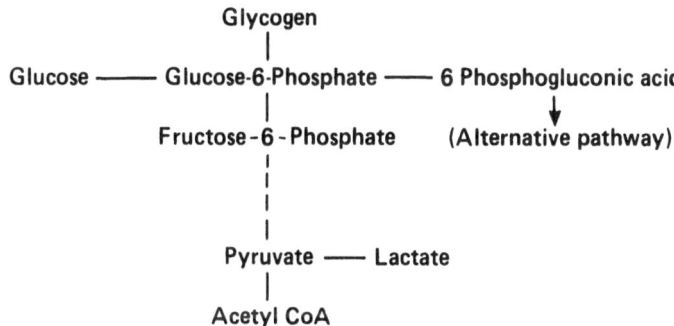

Figure 2.4 The major glycolytic pathway

oxidized NAD for the continuing metabolism of glucose and ATP production. Subsequently when oxygen becomes available lactate is released by muscle tissue and transported to the liver where it is converted via pyruvate to glucose. This is known as the Cori cycle, and it requires energy.

(b) The alternative pathway: hexose monophosphate shunt

This also occurs in the cytoplasm. It involves many intermediates and enzymes which are found in high concentration in the liver and red blood cells. It serves two functions:

- The production of NADPH which plays an important role in fat metabolism and which prevents the accumulation of toxic metabolites such as H_2O_2
- The production of intermediates necessary for nucleic acid synthesis

In summary the majority of glucose is metabolized via the glycolytic pathway to pyruvate. This is then further metabolized through the tricarboxylic acid cycle to carbon dioxide and water. Alternatively in hypoxia pyruvate is converted to lactate which is recycled to glucose in the liver.

(c) Gluconeogenesis

Glucose may be released by the breakdown of storage forms e.g. glycogenolysis, or it may be synthesized by other substances, for example amino acids, by gluconeogenesis. Amino acid metabolism is discussed in Sections 2.4.4 and 2.5.1.

2.4.3 LIPID METABOLISM

(a) Fatty acid oxidation

Most lipid is in the form of triglyceride in fat depots where hydrolysis produces glycerol and fatty acids. Glycerol may enter the glycolytic pathway. The liberated fatty acids are taken up by the mitochondria and undergo a series of enzyme oxidations. Fatty acids with even numbers of carbon atoms enter the tricarboxylic acid cycle via acetyl CoA, whereas those with odd numbers of carbon atoms enter the cycle through propionyl and succinyl CoA, a process which involves Vitamin B12. Long chain fatty acids require carnitine for mitochondrial penetration, but this does not apply to the short chain derivatives.

Where there is an inadequate supply of oxaloacetate, some of which is derived from pyruvate, the acetyl CoA produced from fatty acid metabolism cannot be completely oxidized. This occurs with a high rate of fatty acid oxidation which develops during starvation, with high fat diets, and in uncontrolled diabetes mellitus. Under these circumstances excess acetyl CoA leads to the production of ketone bodies in the liver. Examples include acetoacetate and beta hydroxybutyrate. Extrahepatic tissues oxidize ketone bodies as energy substrates.

(b) Fatty acid synthesis

Fatty acid synthesis occurs predominantly in the cytoplasm. The first and rate limiting step is the synthesis of malonyl CoA from acetyl CoA by acetyl CoA carboxylase which is activated by citrate and inhibited by the products of synthesis. The chains of short chain fatty acids are lengthened in the mitochondria.

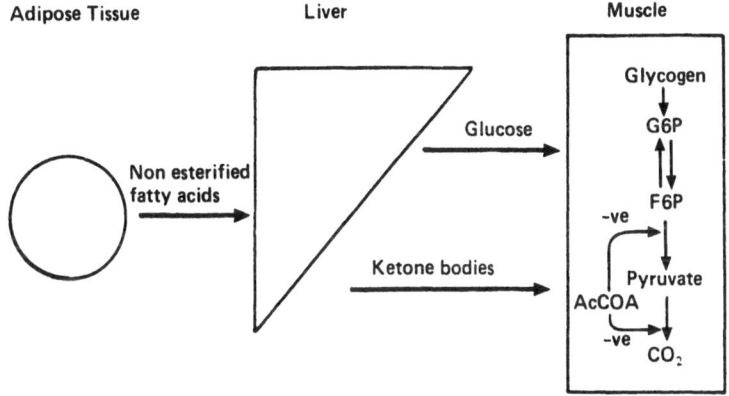

Figure 2.5 Relationship between glucose and lipid metabolism

(Adapted from Smith, R. and Williamson, D. H. (1983) Nutrition: Biochemical Background. In *Oxford Textbook of Medicine*, Weatherall, D. J., Ledingham, J. G. G., Warrell, G. A., (eds) Oxford University Press. 8.4–8.12.)

(c) Interactions between glucose and lipid metabolism

There are important relationships between lipid and glucose metabolism. Increased concentrations of ketone bodies which commonly occur during starvation inhibit glucose utilization by muscle. The mechanism by which this occurs is illustrated in Fig. 2.5. Enhanced fatty acid oxidation leads to increased acetyl CoA production which inhibits:

- Phosphofructokinase thus reducing glycolysis, and
- Pyruvate dehydrogenase

Consequently much of the pyruvate and lactate which is formed can be returned to the liver for conversion to glucose (Cori cycle). The preservation of glucose reduces the need for gluconeogenesis during prolonged starvation and thus preserves muscle protein.

Conversely in the presence of adequate glycogen and glucose, from the diet or gluconeogenesis, acetyl CoA is used for the synthesis of fatty acids. The malonyl CoA thus formed inhibits the enzymes which are responsible for mitochondrial fatty acid uptake. This reduces fatty acid oxidation and encourages esterification.

2.4.4 PROTEIN AND AMINO ACID METABOLISM

There is continual breakdown and resynthesis of body protein equivalent to at least 250 g of muscle tissue each day. Proteins are reduced to their amino acid constituents and these have the general formula shown in Fig. 2.6. There are 20 amino acids in the human body, of which nine are considered essential because they cannot be adequately synthesized. The essential amino acids are discussed in Chapter 3.

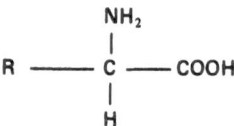

Figure 2.6 General formula of amino acids

(a) Amino acid metabolism

Amino acids participate in numerous metabolic pathways some of which will be summarized.

(i) Deamination Under the influence of enzymes known as transaminases the amino group is transferred to pyruvate or alpha oxoglutarate resulting in the formation of alanine or glutamate:

$$\text{Amino acid} + \text{pyruvate} = \text{keto acid} + \text{alanine}$$

This process is called transamination. The amino group on glutamate can be converted further to ammonia:

$$\text{Glutamate} = \text{alpha ketoglutarate} + NH_3$$

This reaction is termed oxidative deamination.

(ii) Metabolism of the carbon skeleton of amino acids Following deamination the carbon skeleton can enter the pathways of oxidative metabolism. Thirteen amino acids are glycogenic, and their carbon skeletons can be metabolized to tricarboxylic acid cycle intermediates in the liver or kidney. Five are glycogenic or ketogenic, being converted to tricarboxylic acid cycle intermediates or to acetyl CoA.

(iii) The formation of urea   The ammonia produced by oxidative deamination is converted in the liver to urea prior to excretion. This process involves the urea cycle which is illustrated in Fig. 2.7.

There have been reports of high blood ammonia values in infants treated by parenteral nutrition. This has been attributed to the relatively low content of arginine in some crystalline amino acid solutions and has been resolved by arginine supplementation.

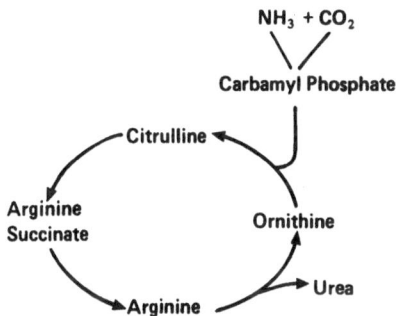

Figure 2.7 Summary of the urea cycle

(iv) Oxidation of branch chain amino acids   The branch chain amino acids are leucine, isoleucine and valine. After ingestion there is minimal uptake in the liver as they are metabolized in skeletal muscle. Leucine is thought to stimulate muscle protein synthesis. For these reasons branch chain enriched amino acid solutions are under evaluation in hypercatabolic patients in an attempt to reduce muscle wasting. Preliminary reports have failed to provide convincing evidence that such solutions will achieve this objective.

(v) The glucose-alanine cycle   Alanine is mainly produced from pyruvate by the transamination of amino acids, particularly glutamate. Glutamate is a product of branch chain amino acid metabolism and pyruvate is derived from glycolysis in the liver. The glucose alanine cycle is illustrated in Fig. 2.8.

This cycle serves to dispose of amino groups from various amino acids in the form of urea. In this way alanine plays an important role in gluconeogenesis. In short-term starvation and uncontrolled diabetes mellitus, alanine is derived from proteolysis and pyruvate from the

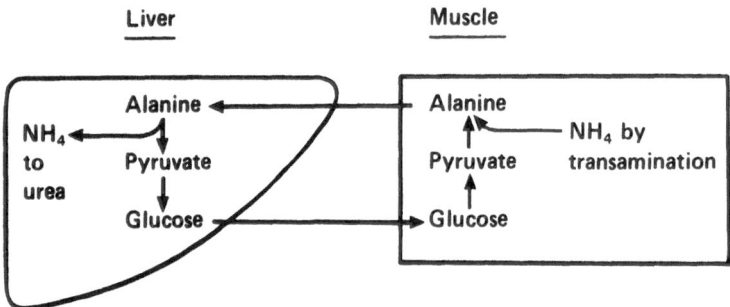

Figure 2.8 The glucose alanine cycle

(Adapted from Smith, R. and Williamson, D. H. (1983) Nutrition: Biochemical Background. In *Oxford Textbook of Medicine*, Weatherall, D. J., Ledingham, J. G. G., Warrell, G. A., (eds) Oxford University Press. 8.4–8.12.)

partial oxidation of other amino acids. This process is reduced during prolonged starvation.

(b) Protein synthesis

The basis of protein synthesis is the reaction of the carboxyl group of one amino acid with the amino group of another. The amino acids concerned are first joined to the template RNA in the ribosome of the cytoplasm. The RNA determines the amino acid sequence and the RNA structure is in turn fashioned on the nuclear DNA.

This is an energy-dependent process which leads to the formation of peptide chains, the amino acid sequence of which determines their three-dimensional structure. Thus proteins are coded by DNA and built via RNA.

2.4.5 MICRONUTRIENT METABOLISM

Micronutrients include trace elements and vitamins and play an important role in metabolic processes. These functions will be reviewed. The sources and requirements of micronutrients are discussed in Chapter 3, and micronutrient deficiency syndromes are described in Chapter 4.

(a) Trace element and mineral metabolism

Iron serves two major functions. Iron atoms in haemoglobin and myoglobin combine reversibly with oxygen for its transport and supply. Iron facilitaties electron transfer in the cytoplasm of all cells for oxidation reactions during intermediary metabolism. Zinc forms part of at least 80 metalloenzymes and plays a role in the synthesis of proteins, DNA and RNA. Manganese activates many enzymes and stimulates RNA and DNA polymerase activity.

Fluoride protects against dental caries. Copper is found in a number of metalloenzymes and participates in oxidation and reduction reactions. Trivalent chromium is a component of nucleic acids and glucose tolerance factor which facilitates the interreaction of glucose and its receptors. Hexavalent chromium is toxic.

Selenium is an integral part of the enzyme glutathione peroxidase and is required for the efficient oxidation of sulphydryl groups. Selenium and Vitamin E are both involved in maintaining a low intracellular concentration of potentially harmful free radicals. Iodide is concentrated in the thyroid gland for thyroid hormone synthesis and cobalt is a component of Vitamin B12.

Finally the more common minerals participate in important metabolic functions. Phosphate is involved in cellular energy metabolism and acid secretion. Calcium is concerned with neuromuscular function and is particularly important in cardiac muscle. Magnesium is involved in ATP dependent reactions, protein synthesis, and neuromuscular transmission and activity. It is required for parathyroid hormone secretion and receptor activity, and many of the other symptoms of magnesium deficiency are attributable to secondary hypocalcaemia.

(b) Vitamin metabolism

Vitamins are important coenzymes in fat carbohydrate and protein metabolism; examples of metabolic functions of some water soluble vitamins are given in Table 2.6. The tricarboxylic acid cycle requires coenzymes which are formed from nicotinic acid, riboflavin, thiamin, pantothenic acid, biotin and pyridoxine. Thiamin is involved in the metabolism of carbohydrates, alcohol and branch chain amino acids. Vitamin A is required for the integrity of mucus-secreting epithelia and mucopolysaccharide synthesis. Vitamin C is important in connective tissue metabolism; it also facilitates iron absorption from vegetable foods and it inhibits nitrosamine formation. This may explain the epidemiological observation of an inverse relationship between Vitamin C ingestion and gastric cancer. Vitamin B12 and folate are involved in purine metabolism. Vitamin K is employed in the hepatic synthesis of coagulation factors. Vitamin D has an important role in mineral metabolism. This vitamin, which

Table 2.6 Examples of metabolic functions of some water soluble vitamins

Vitamin	Function
Thiamin (B1)	Aerobic decarboxylation
Riboflavin (B2)	Oxidation. Reduction
Pyridoxine (B6)	Transamination. Decarboxylation
Pantothenic Acid	Metabolism of fatty acids
Biotin	Carboxylation. Decarboxylation

is either ingested or formed in the skin by the action of sunlight on 7 dehydrocholesterol, is first converted to 25 hydroxy Vitamin D in the liver and subsequently to 1,25 dihydroxy Vitamin D in the kidney. The latter is the active component which primarily promotes intestinal calcium absorption.

2.5 Response to starvation and injury

When nutrient intake is interrupted there is an immediate need to provide essential nutrients such as glucose from tissue stores to fuel metabolic processes. This is followed by metabolic adaption for the conservation of vital tissues and the utilization of fat depots, unless the patient is stressed by sepsis or trauma. Under these circumstances the overriding priority is enhanced provision of energy substrate and amino acids for tissue repair and hepatic protein synthesis. In practice the natural history of disease dictates that many patients are initially starved and subsequently stressed. Examples include patients with Crohn's disease or intestinal neoplasia when surgery may be required after a period of under-nutrition or malabsorption.

2.5.1 STARVATION

(a) Acute starvation

The central nervous system, haemopoietic system and renal medulla require glucose as an energy substrate. There is an obligatory daily need for 150–250 g of glucose. The liver derives its energy from fatty acids or ketone body metabolism. Other tissues such as skeletal muscle can use glucose and fatty acids or ketones as energy sources.

Relatively little glucose is available from glycogenolysis because of the limited supply of hepatic glycogen. Most is initially produced by gluconeogenesis which occurs mainly in the kidney and liver.

The main substrate for gluconeogenesis in the kidney is glutamine which is derived from the transamination of other amino acids. In the liver it is alanine, much of which is produced by the transamination of branch chain amino acids in the muscle and which participates in the glucose alanine cycle (see Fig. 2.8). Lipolysis provides fatty acids to fuel hepatic metabolism.

(b) Prolonged starvation

During prolonged starvation many fundamental metabolic changes occur. These are summarized in Fig. 2.9. Reduced insulin concentra-

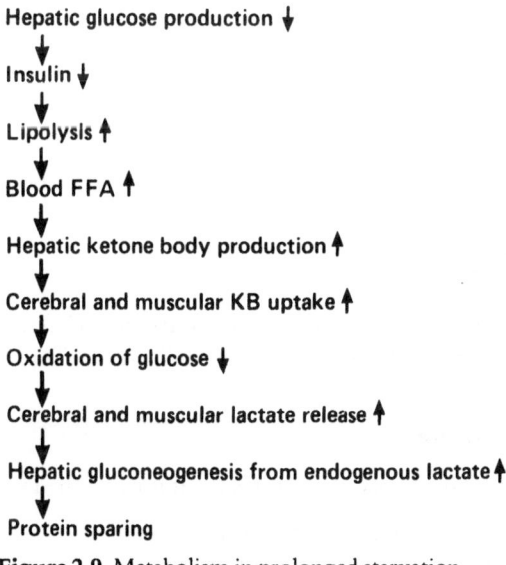

Hepatic glucose production ↓
↓
Insulin ↓
↓
Lipolysis ↑
↓
Blood FFA ↑
↓
Hepatic ketone body production ↑
↓
Cerebral and muscular KB uptake ↑
↓
Oxidation of glucose ↓
↓
Cerebral and muscular lactate release ↑
↓
Hepatic gluconeogenesis from endogenous lactate ↑
↓
Protein sparing

Figure 2.9 Metabolism in prolonged starvation

Table 2.7 The metabolic response to starvation

Basal metabolic rate	Reduced
Hormonal changes	Small increase followed by reduced secretion of cortisol catecholamines, growth hormone and glucagon. Insulin decreased
Energy source	Initially protein and fat, subsequently fat
Nitrogen	Losses decrease
Electrolytes	Initial loss. Subsequent conservation

tion permits increased lipolysis, and tissues including the central nervous system adapt to the metabolism of ketone bodies. The formation of glucose from protein is reduced, the glucose which is formed is oxidized to a lesser extent and is released more often in the form of lactate which may be re-used in the Cori cycle (see Section 2.4.2). Ketone body metabolism is regulated by two mechanisms, the insulotrophic properties of ketone bodies and their direct inhibitory effect on adipose tissue lipolysis.

In this way fat is utilized and protein is conserved. The metabolic response to starvation is summarized in Table 2.7.

2.5.2 INJURY

Classical teaching describes three phases in the metabolic response to injury.

(a) The ebb phase

This is transient, lasting only a few hours. It is characterized by the secretion of catecholamines and the mobilization of hepatic glycogen.

(b) The flow phase

This may last for many days or weeks. It is concerned with:

- The maintenance of energy production
- The provision of substrate for protein synthesis and tissue repair

It is characterized by an increase in catecholamines, glucagon, cortisol and growth hormone. Whereas insulin values are also increased there is relative insulin resistance. There is breakdown of both protein and fat with increased nitrogen losses and sodium retention. The metabolic rate increases.

During this phase the restoration of a positive nitrogen balance by aggressive nutritional support is always difficult, usually impossible and frequently hazardous. Nutritional therapy aims to minimize losses and replace essential nutrients until the stress-inducing factors have been treated and removed. The over-provision of energy and nitrogen in an attempt to replace all losses may impose further metabolic stress. It has recently been recognized that glucose tolerance is limited in stressed patients and overall energy needs are not as high as previously thought. Few patients need more than 2000 kcal (8.4 MJ) per day, half of which should be given as lipid. The use of more dextrose will simply lead to steatosis. This is not only metabolically inefficient, but it also generates carbon dioxide and consumes oxygen imposing increased respiratory demands. This subject is discussed further in Chapters 6 and 7.

(c) The anabolic phase

The anabolic phase lasts for a variable period depending on the type of injury. There is restoration of depleted tissue at a maximum rate in a 70 kg male of 3–5 g of nitrogen per day. In practice this phase takes longer than predicted because optimum anabolism is not initially achieved or subsequently maintained.

The difficulties posed by the nutritional support of stressed patients serve to emphasize the need where possible to correct malnutrition associated with starvation before subjecting a patient to the potential stress of surgery and its sequelae.

2.5.3 THE REGULATION OF SUBSTRATE METABOLISM

(a) Endocrine regulation

The endocrine regulation of substrate metabolism is summarized in Fig. 2.10. In the presence of anabolic hormones substrates are stored in depots, whereas the catabolic hormones encourage sub-

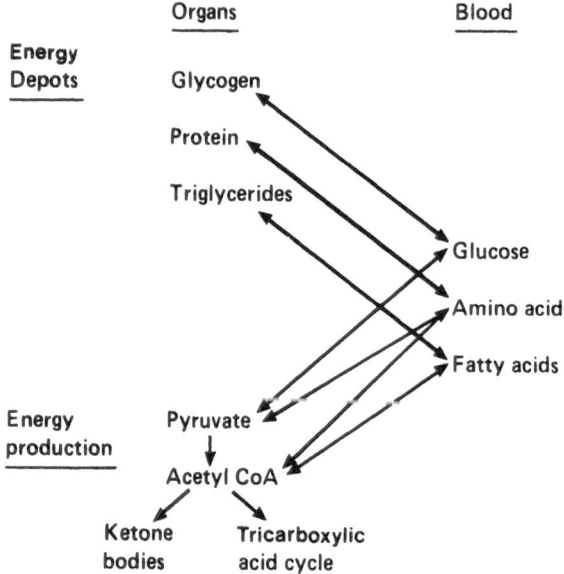

Figure 2.10 Endocrine regulation of substrate metabolism

Table 2.8 Hormones and substrate metabolism

Anabolic hormones	Catabolic hormones
Insulin	Catecholamines
Growth hormone	Glucocorticoids
Androgens	Glucagon

strate mobilization. The major hormones involved with substrate catabolism are shown in Table 2.8.

(i) Anabolic hormones Insulin is the main anabolic hormone and it has many functions. It increases glucose uptake, amino acid uptake and glycogen, fatty acid and triglyceride synthesis. It decreases amino acid metabolism, gluconeogenesis and fatty acid oxidation.

Growth hormone stimulates nitrogen, phosphorus and potassium retention, but it induces lipolysis and ketogenesis. Androgens play a relatively minor role in this context.

(ii) Catabolic hormones   Catecholamines are released early in response to stress. They stimulate glycogenolysis, gluconeogenesis, lipolysis and amino acid release. They depress insulin secretion.

Glucocorticoids inhibit protein synthesis and mobilize fatty acids. However they enhance the formation of fat and glycogen. They also suppress insulin secretion, and enhance glucagon release.

Glucagon induces gluconeogenesis, glycogenolysis, proteolysis, and lipolysis.

(b) Humeral factors

Factors such as leukocyte endogenous mediator which are under prostaglandin control may be isolated from the plasma of seriously ill patients. They induce muscle proteolysis and encourage the synthesis of specific proteins by the liver.

2.6 Digestion and absorption

Food contains complex molecules of carbohydrate, fat and protein, as well as minerals, vitamins and water. Prior to absorption food must be broken down into simple components by the process of digestion under the influence of various intestinal and pancreatic enzymes. Fig. 2.11 summarizes the sources of the most important enzymes and the main sites of absorption. The important steps in the digestion and absorption of the major dietary components will now be discussed.

2.6.1 CARBOHYDRATE

Carbohydrate is largely composed of starch, sucrose and lactose, but the many forms of carbohydrate include cellulose and other components of the cell wall which cannot be broken down in humans and are described as dietary fibre. Starch is a glucose polymer consisting of amylose with alpha 1–4 links and amylopectin in which there are alpha 1–4 links and alpha 1–6 cross-links.

The digestion and absorption of carbohydrate involve three stages: luminal hydrolysis, mucosal hydrolysis and mucosal transport.

(a) Luminal hydrolysis

Hydrolysis is begun by salivary amylase the activity of which is reduced by the low gastric pH. It is continued by pancreatic amylase.

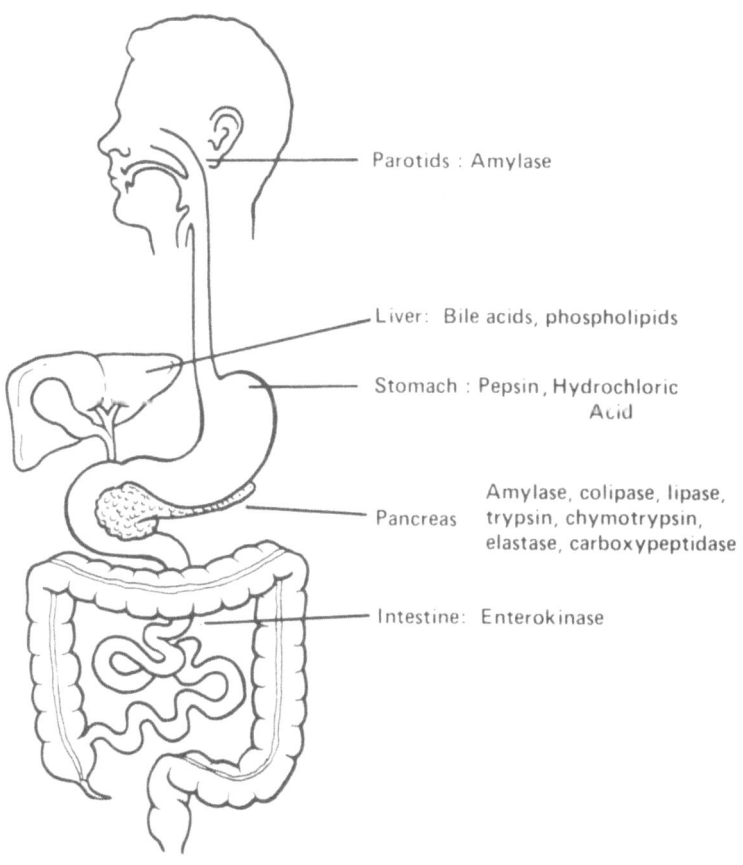

Figure 2.11 Anatomy of the digestive tract

These enzymes hydrolyse alpha 1–4 bonds, but not those at the end of polymer chains or adjacent to alpha 1–6 bonds. Starch is thus degraded to maltose, maltotriose, and five to eight molecule glucose polymers containing alpha 1–4 and alpha 1–6 bonds. Very little glucose is produced.

(b) Mucosal hydrolysis

Many brush border enzymes, for example glucoamylase, sucrase, maltase and lactase, effect mucosal hydrolysis, liberating mono saccharides such as glucose and galactose. Feedback inhibition prevents the build-up of monosaccharides which would be osmotically disadvantageous.

Some individuals are deficient in enzymes, usually lactase. Lactase activity may be reduced in various forms of small intestinal disease. Under these circumstances unhydrolysed lactose acts as an osmotic purgative. Consequently most commercially available enteral feeds contain little or no lactose.

(c) Mucosal transport

Glucose and galactose are transported by an active carrier system which is driven by the diffusion of sodium down the concentration gradient. ATP is subsequently required to pump sodium out of the cell. Consequently commercially available rehydration solutions are isotonic with equimolar concentrations of glucose and sodium facilitating water and electrolyte absorption.

Fructose enters the mucosal cell by facilitated diffusion. A similar process governs the transfer of monosaccharides from the cell to the portal blood in which they are transported for hepatic metabolism.

2.6.2 FAT

Normal individuals have a large absorptive reserve of at least four times the average fat consumption. Dietary fat is mostly in the form of triglycerides (see Fig. 2.1) with long chain fatty acids. Some fatty acids of vegetable origin have double bonds so are unsaturated, but this does not influence digestion or absorption. Medium chain triglycerides with 8–12 carbon atoms are water soluble and are absorbed differently.

(a) Intraluminal phase

Emulsification is achieved by gastric motility and enhanced by biliary and dietary phospholipids, and to a lesser extent by bile acids. Lipolysis is primarily effected by pancreatic lipase and colipase at the 1 and 3 positions. In neonates lingual and gastric lipases are more active and have a predilection for medium chain triglycerides.

Following emulsification and lipolysis the monoglycerides and free fatty acids along with cholesterol and fat soluble vitamins are rendered water soluble in the form of micelles by the presence of bile acids. Bile acids are synthesized in the liver from cholesterol with hydrophobic end chains and they surround the lipid products.

(b) Membrane phase

The idea that pinocytosis engulfs the micelle is no longer tenable. Lipids diffuse passively across the cell membrane and the bile acids return to the intestinal lumen for participation in further micelle formation prior to active absorption via the specialized epithelium of the terminal ileum.

(c) Enterocyte phase

Fatty acids are bound by fatty acid binding protein in the cytosol. They are actively re-esterified in the smooth endoplasmic reticulum. This process maintains concentration gradients favouring further absorption. Lipoproteins and phospholipids are also synthesized in the endoplasmic reticulum and form chylomicrons with triglycerides. The chylomicrons are discharged into the lymphatics by reverse pinocytosis.

(d) Medium chain triglycerides

Medium chain triglycerides are water soluble. They can diffuse through the enterocyte into venous tributaries of the portal system. This has relevance for nutritional practice. Fat is provided in this form for patients in whom the mechanisms of fat digestion and absorption are significantly impaired.

2.6.3 PROTEIN

(a) Intraluminal phase

Hydrolysis of protein molecules occurs at the internal CO–NH bonds in the peptide chain. This is facilitated by:

- Gastric pepsins which produce medium and long chain poly-peptides
- Pancreatic enzymes which include trypsin, chymotrypsin,

elastase and carboxypeptidase which are excreted in inactive form. Intestinal enterokinase converts inactive trypsinogen to trypsin which activates the other enzymes

Hydrolysis in the lumen of the duodenum and proximal jejunum produces free amino acids and peptide chains of two to six amino acids in length.

(b) Mucosal phase

There are two fundamental mechanisms of mucosal absorption:

- The transport of free amino acids by group specific transport systems
- The separate uptake of short chain peptides

The latter mechanism appears to have a distinct kinetic advantage. This has implications for nutritional support. The use of peptide solutions may improve absorption and reduce the nutrient osmolality, and are thus preferred in patients with maldigestion and impaired absorption.

2.6.4 MINERAL AND ELECTROLYTE ABSORPTION

Mineral absorption is affected by luminal factors, mucosal function and extraneous influences such as ethanol and hormonal and endocrine status.

(a) Luminal factors

High fibre diets may impair the absorption of calcium and zinc. Binding occurs with uronic acids derived from cellulose, and phytate. This may be reduced with high protein diets, since protein hydrolysis releases fibre bound zinc.

Diseases which are accompanied by steatorrhoea are associated with reduced absorption of calcium and magnesium which form insoluble soaps with long chain fatty acids. Under these circumstances magnesium and calcium loss can be reduced by substituting medium chain triglycerides, the salts of which are more soluble.

A high calcium intake may lower magnesium absorption. This can result in hypomagnesaemia in neonates fed on cow's milk. Alcohol reduces the absorption of divalent ions and greatly increases the urinary excretion of magnesium. Drugs such as Oxytetracycline form insoluble complexes with iron.

(b) Mucosal phase

(i) Minerals Calcium is absorbed by active and passive processes. Active transport mechanisms exist for iron and zinc, but magnesium is probably absorbed passively. Iron is absorbed in the duodenum and proximal jejunum, and other minerals are absorbed throughout the small intestine. Iron deficiency is characteristic of mucosal disease such as gluten enteropathy which maximally affects the proximal small intestine.

Mucosal uptake is also influenced by other factors. The absorption of both iron and magnesium is increased in deficiency states and calcium absorption is dependent upon Vitamin D status.

(ii) Electrolytes Electrolyte absorption occurs partly by passive absorption with water following osmotic and hydrostatic gradients. The aqueous channels are negatively charged and thus cation selective. They are tighter in the ileum and especially in the colon where absorption is slower and so solvent drag is less important. Diseases such as gluten enteropathy are associated with reduced pore size, so consequently absorption may also be reduced. Specific carrier mechanisms also exist. Sodium shares active transport with glucose and amino acids in the jejunum. A sodium-hydrogen exchange pump occurs throughout the small intestine, and is favoured by luminal bicarbonate which reduces the concentration gradient of excreted hydrogen. There is also a separate electrogenic mechanism. Sodium which is absorbed into the enterocyte is actively extruded by a sodium-potassium exchange pump at the baso-lateral border.

Approximately nine litres of fluid and 1500 mmol of sodium enter the intestine each day. Only 1.5 litres are ingested, and the remainder is produced in the gastrointestinal and biliary secretions. There is normally a large reserve for fluid and electrolyte absorption, and estimates suggest a capacity for the absorption of 15–20 litres of isotonic saline.

2.6.5 VITAMINS

The fat soluble Vitamins A, D, and K are incorporated into micelles and diffuse passively across the small intestinal mucosa. The metabolite of Vitamin D, 25 hydroxy Vitamin D, subsequently participates in an enteropathic circulation via the terminal ileum.

Absorption of Vitamin C is by an active sodium-dependent mechanism which is confined to the ileum, although passive absorption of large doses may occur by diffusion. Thiamin is absorbed in the proximal jejunum, and the absorption of thiamin, niacin and biotin involves active transport mechanisms. The absorption of riboflavin is facilitated by bile acids.

Folate is absorbed in the duodenum and proximal jejunum. Vitamin B12 is actively absorbed in the terminal ileum after binding with the glycoprotein intrinsic factor which is synthesized in the stomach.

2.7 Intestinal adaption

2.7.1 THE EFFECTS OF INTESTINAL RESECTION

The normal intestine has a large functional reserve and half the length can be removed with no subsequent major problems. Patients can survive with very little residual intestine because of adaption by the remaining bowel.

Whereas most nutrients are absorbed in the proximal small intestine, the loss of which will additionally reduce cholecystokinin and thus pancreatic and biliary secretions, more problems are posed by ileal resection. This is because the ileum absorbs bile acids as well as Vitamin B12 and 25 hydroxy Vitamin D. The colonic bacterial degradation of bile acids produces toxic metabolites which induce electrolyte secretion. The loss of less than 100 cm of ileum will cause diarrhoea but no significant steatorrhoea. Larger resections will also cause steatorrhoea. Loss of the ileo-caecal valve compounds the problem by reducing intestinal transit time and facilitating intestinal colonization. Patients who also have colonic disease usually suffer more severe diarrhoea.

Intestinal adaption involves an increase in bowel length and villus height. It is much greater in the ileum after jejunal resection than in the jejunum after ileal resection. Functional adaption accompanies structural change with increased absorption of carbohydrate, fat and amino acids per unit length. Adaption commences within a few days of resection provided luminal nutrition is available.

2.7.2 THE MECHANISM OF INTESTINAL ADAPTION

Three major factors facilitate intestinal adaption.

(a) Luminal nutrition

This is essential, so enteral nutrition must be provided following resection. However, there is evidence that with malnutrition adaption occurs more rapidly when enteral nutrition is supplemented with parenteral nutrition. Furthermore long chain fatty acids appear particularly important, whereas medium chain triglycerides are less effective in the induction of adaption.

These patients who all initially suffer from malabsorption are frequently fed enteral feeds containing medium chain triglycerides which are better tolerated. Fibre is said to facilitate colonic adaption.

(b) Pancreatic and biliary secretions

Pancreatic secretions in particular appear to enhance adaption.

(c) Enteric hormones

Many hormones may have a role in promoting intestinal adaption. Enteroglucagon appears to be particularly important. It is found in the distal small intestine and colon, and is released in response to fat or carbohydrate which escapes absorption in the proximal small bowel. It promotes mucosal growth and slows intestinal transit.

2.8 Water and electrolyte metabolism

2.8.1 DISTRIBUTION OF WATER AND ELECTROLYTES

As discussed in Section 2.1 a 70 kg male contains 40 litres of water distributed between the intracellular and extracellular spaces (see Fig. 2.2). Sodium is the predominant cation in the extracellular component, and potassium predominates in the intracellular component (see Table 2.5).

The extracellular fluid can be subdivided into the interstitial fluid in which the protein concentration is very low and the intravascular fluid which contains the plasma proteins. The distribution of water in these compartments is governed by osmotic and hydrostatic pressures which act in opposing directions. The total body water is regulated by the variable permeability of the renal tubules under the influence of antidiuretic hormone.

The distribution of water between the cells and extracellular fluid is mainly influenced by osmotic forces in which sodium is particularly important. Because cell membranes are permeable sodium and potassium concentration gradients are maintained by energy-dependent pumps.

2.8.2 WATER AND ELECTROLYTE BALANCE

The factors influencing water balance are summarized in Table 2.9.

Table 2.9 Factors influencing water balance

Input	Output
Liquids	Urine
Solid food	Faecal water
Metabolic water	Evaporation*

*Includes loss through the skin and respiratory tract

(a) Fluid intake

Fluids are drunk by social habit and thirst is an additional physiological regulating mechanism. The sensation of thirst arises when small increases in osmolarity stimulate thirst centres in the hypothalamus. This responds primarily to water depletion: patients who are febrile and sweat profusely may be salt and water depleted with no complaint of thirst. The amount of fluid ingested is variable depending on individual circumstances. Most people drink 1.5 – 2 litres per day.

The water content of food, and water produced by metabolism, both depend on diet. The metabolism of 1 g of starch, protein and fat respectively yields 0.6, 0.4, and 1 g of water. Metabolic water will often contribute 400 ml per day.

(b) Fluid output

Each day approximately nine litres of water and 1500 mmol of sodium are secreted into the gastrointestinal tract, and 200 litres of water and 3000 mmol of sodium are filtered through the glomerulus. Consequently abnormalities of gastrointestinal or renal function readily lead to water and electrolyte depletion. Normally net daily losses amount to 100 ml of water and 15 mmol of sodium in the faeces and 1.5 litres and 100 mmol of sodium in the urine.

Urine losses vary widely, being largely determined by the volume of ingested fluid. The minimum necessary volume is that which is required to excrete the obligatory solute load. With normal renal function the maximum urine concentration is 1200 m osm/kg. This implies the need for 0.5–1 litre of urine with an average diet. The failure to ingest sufficient water to meet this need will lead to impaired renal function and urea retention. Much larger volumes will be required in patients with renal impairment. Larger volumes will also need to be secreted by hypercatabolic patients receiving hyper-alimentation.

The normal kidney is able to conserve sodium so that as little as 2–3 mmol a day may be excreted. Renal impairment may lead to the inability to excrete sodium with diseases such as glomerulonephritis which are associated with reduced glomerular filtration rate, or inability to conserve sodium with distal tubular disease as in analgesic nephropathy or pyelonephritis. Because sodium and potassium are exchanged across the distal tubule and sodium is conserved preferentially the obligatory potassium loss is greater, approximately 20–30 mmol per day.

Normally 900 mmol of fluid are lost by evaporation from the respiratory tract and skin. Disorders associated with hyperventilation such as pneumonia will increase respiratory losses. Pyrexial patients may sweat profusely and can lose 1–2 litres of fluid a day. It is important to note that each litre of sweat contains 20–80 mmol of sodium and 5–15 mmol of potassium.

(c) Fluid balance

In summary, daily insensible losses, water lost from the skin and respiratory tract minus the metabolic water production amounts to 500 ml. A further 100 ml may be lost in the faeces and there is a minimum requirement of 900 ml for urinary secretion. Thus under normal circumstances there is a minimum daily need for 1.5 litres of water. However it must be remembered that these figures are variable and much greater losses will be sustained by most patients.

2.8.3 REGULATION OF WATER AND ELECTROLYTE METABOLISM

The body content of water and electrolytes is determined by extracellular concentration.

(a) Control of electrolytes

Sodium retention is influenced by:

- Renal function: a reduced glomerular infiltration rate promotes sodium retention and abnormal function leads to sodium loss
- Aldosterone which promotes sodium retention in exchange for potassium across cell membranes
- Naturetic hormone which reduces sodium reabsorption in the proximal renal tubule in response to expansion of the plasma volume

In health aldosterone plays a major role in controlling sodium status. Reduction of the blood volume leads to reduced renal perfusion and this in turn stimulates renin secretion from the juxtaglomerular apparatus in the renal cortex. Renin is a proteolytic enzyme which acts on an alpha 2 globulin to form angiotensin 1 which is further split to angiotensin 2. This leads to vasoconstriction and aldosterone secretion by the zona glomerulosa in the adrenal cortex.

(b) Control of water

An increase in plasma osmolality which is normally predominantly determined by sodium concentration has two effects:

- An increase in water intake via the hypothalamic thirst centre
- A reduction in renal water excretion by the pituitary release of antidiuretic hormone which facilitates water reabsorption through the renal tubule

Thus changes in plasma volume govern sodium retention and changes in plasma osmolality, reflecting sodium concentration, influence water retention.

2.8.4 DISTURBANCE OF WATER AND ELECTROLYTE BALANCE

(a) Depletion of water and electrolytes

Pure deficiency or excess of sodium or water is rare. Water depletion often accompanies sodium loss, and potassium balance is related to the acid-base status. The clinical features of water and electrolyte imbalance will be discussed in Chapter 4.

(i) Predominant water depletion   This occurs with either excessive fluid loss due to gastroenteritis and sweat or due to deficiency of fluid intake in the patient who is unconscious or who has oesophageal disease. Rarely water depletion is due to the failure of homeostatic mechanisms as in diabetes insipidus: a deficiency of ADH or the failure of renal response to this hormone.

(ii) Predominant sodium depletion   Predominant sodium depletion occurs with vomiting, diarrhoea, fistulous loss or excessive sweating which is followed by replacement with fluids containing insufficient sodium. Sodium depletion occasionally develops due to the failure of homeostatic mechanisms as in Addison's disease with the loss of aldosterone, and sodium losing renal disease.

Because of the relationship between sodium and water the sodium status is not reflected by changes in plasma sodium concentration. Sodium and water depletion has to be judged clinically on the basis of skin turgor, blood pressure and urine flow. When severe it will lead to haemoconcentration and uraemia.

(iii) Potassium depletion   Potassium depletion occurs when there is inadequate intake because renal potassium conservation is not as efficient as that for sodium. Depletion is particularly likely to occur through the loss of intestinal secretions in patients who vomit or have intestinal fistulae or diarrhoea. Increased renal losses accompany renal tubular failure (when increased urinary sodium is available for exchange across the distal tubule), and occur during diuretic therapy and in the presence of hyperaldosteronism.

Plasma potassium values do not necessarily reflect body potassium stores. For example, diabetic keto acidosis is typically associated with potassium depletion yet patients are frequently hyperkalaemic at presentation. This is because cells buffer hydrogen in acidotic patients when hydrogen is exchanged for potassium across the cell membrane. Significant deficiency leads to muscle weakness and paralytic ileus.

(b) Water and electrolyte overload

(i) Predominant water excess Predominant water excess occurs in oliguric renal failure where excessive fluid of low sodium content has been administered. It is rarely caused by excessive ADH secretion which prevents water excretion. Such patients may be profoundly hyponatraemic with cerebral oedema which leads to drowsiness and convulsions.

(ii) Primary sodium excess Rarely this is due to endocrine disorders causing excessive secretion of aldosterone (Conn's syndrome) or mineralocorticoids (Cushing's syndrome). It commonly occurs in patients with malnutrition, chronic liver disease and cardiac failure. In many of these patients hypoalbuminaemia reduces the effective plasma volume and thus stimulates aldosterone secretion. The patients may be hypokalaemic because of secondary hyperaldosteronism.

Sodium overload cannot be identified by serum sodium measurements. Patients with endocrine disorders are often hypertensive, and those with malnutrition, hepatic or cardiac disease are oedematous. Both groups may be hypokalaemic.

(iii) Potassium excess This is frequently associated with renal failure and is particularly associated with potassium-sparing diuretics. It may lead to fatal cardiac dysrhythmia.

Careful attention must be paid to the water and electrolyte status. Abnormalities of fluid and electrolyte balance require correction before effective nutritional support can be administered. This is particularly important in patients who require parenteral nutrition.

References

Cahill, G. F. (1976) Starvation in man. *Clinical Endocrinol. Metabolism*, **5**, 397–415.

McGilvery R. W. and Goldstein, G. (1981) *Biochemistry, a Functional Approach.* W. B. Saunders, Philadelphia.

Robinson, A. M. and Williamson, D. M. (1980). Physiological roles of ketone bodies as substrate and as signals in mammalian tissues. *Physiol. Rev.*, **60**, 143–87.

Ruderman, N. B. (1975) Muscle amino acid metabolism and gluconeogenesis. *Ann. Rev. Med.*, **26**, 245–58.

Sodeman, W. A. and Sodeman, T. M. (1985) *Pathologic Physiology: Mechanisms of Disease*, 7th edn, W. B. Saunders, Philadelphia.

3

THE DIET AND NUTRITIONAL REQUIREMENTS

3.1 Food

The food we eat is derived from vegetable, animal and miscellaneous sources.

3.1.1 FOOD OF VEGETABLE ORIGIN

Food of vegetable origin includes cereals, legumes, roots, leaves, fruits and nuts.

(a) Cereals

The common cereals are listed in Table 3.1. The outer layers of the cereal contain most of the fibre and the highest concentrations of vitamins such as thiamin, riboflavin and niacin as well as minerals such as iron and zinc. It therefore follows that refining the cereal by removing the husk reduces the nutritive value as well as the fibre content.

Wheat is the most universally important cereal and its composition is summarized in Table 3.2. Gluten constitutes up to 90% of the protein. Hard wheats are rich in gluten and provide 'strong flour'

Table 3.1   Common cereal foods

Wheat
Rye
Barley
Oats
Rice
Maize
Millet

Table 3.2   The composition of wheat

Starch	70–75%
Protein	7–15%
Lipid	1–2%
Water	14%

which is used for making bread. Wheat is closely related to rye and barley, and for this reason patients with coeliac disease who are intolerant of gluten should also avoid these cereals. Rye is still used to make bread which is rich in fibre and B vitamins. Barley is principally employed in brewing for the production of beer and whisky.

Oats contain more protein and oil than other common cereals, and consumption is mainly in the form of breakfast cereal such as porridge or muesli. Rice is second to wheat in global importance, and although the proportion of protein is relatively less (6–8%) this is of high quality. The introduction of more effective methods of refinement with more complete removal of the outer husk has substantially reduced not only the fibre but also the B vitamin content of this cereal. This is of considerable nutritional importance because rice constitutes such a large part of the diet in many underdeveloped countries.

Maize is an important cereal in parts of Central America and Africa. The principal protein is zein which lacks lysine and tryptophan. This is important in the relationship between maize and pellagra. Yellow maize contains carotenoids which have pro-Vitamin A activity. Millets are cereals characterized by drought resistance and good-quality protein, and they are grown widely in Africa.

(b) Legumes

Legumes include peas, beans, soya beans, lentils and groundnuts. They are a rich source of protein, the methionine content of which is relatively low, and they complement cereals. This combination provides a cheap and nutritious protein diet.

The soya bean contains up to 40% protein and 20% fat. It is an important source of protein in many parts of the world such as China and it is being used increasingly in the West for the production of margarine and milk substitutes. Groundnuts contain 40% fat and they are used to produce oils and margarines.

(c) Root vegetables

Each 100 g of potato includes 70–80 g of water, 20 g of starch and only 2 g of protein. Potatoes contain small amounts of minerals and Vitamins C and B, and they are a rich source of potassium and fibre. Sweet potatoes, yams and cassava also contain much starch, but there is less than 1% by weight of protein in the latter. Less starch is found in carrots, onions, radishes and turnips.

(d) Leaves, fruits and nuts

Leafy vegetables are an important source of beta carotene, Vitamin C and folate. They also supply significant amounts of riboflavin, iron and calcium, although the presence of oxalate may reduce absorption of the latter and much Vitamin C may be lost during food preparation. Fruits are a major source of Vitamin C most of which is available as they are frequently eaten uncooked. Both fruits and vegetables supply fibre. Nuts have a high fat and protein content, but they are eaten in relatively small quantities and so they make an insignificant dietary contribution.

3.1.2 FOOD OF ANIMAL ORIGIN

Foods of animal origin include meat, fish, eggs, milk and cheese.

(a) Meat

Protein in meat is of high biological value, being rich in essential amino acids. The energy content depends on the amount of associated fat. Meat is an important source of iron and zinc, nicotinic acid and riboflavin, but it contains little calcium, Vitamin A or Vitamin C. Most meats contain a moderate amount of Vitamin B12 which is concentrated in the liver.

(b) Fish

Fish protein is also of high biological value and fish is an important source of iodide and fluoride. Fish oils contain high concentrations of Vitamin A and Vitamin D.

(c) Eggs

Egg protein, much of which is in the form of albumen in the egg white, has a very high biological value and is used as a standard by which other proteins are compared. Eggs contain significant amounts of thiamin, nicotinic acid and riboflavin, and are also rich in cholesterol. The iron content is poorly absorbed because of binding by protein.

(d) Milk, cheese and butter

In addition to high-quality protein, of which there is more in cow's milk than human milk, milk contains carbohydrate in the form of lactose and a variable amount of fat. The calcium content is high and milk also contains small amounts of iron, Vitamin D and Vitamin C.

Cheese contains a variable amount of fat and other nutrients such as calcium and Vitamin A in addition to milk protein. Butter has a high fat content with fat soluble vitamins particularly Vitamin A. The butter substitute margarine is fortified with Vitamins A and D and is made of polyunsaturated fat.

3.1.3 MISCELLANEOUS FOODS

Miscellaneous foods include refined sugar and honey. These provide energy without other nutrients, and excessive consumption contributes to the problems of obesity and dental caries. Drinks and beverages may also have a significant influence on nutritional status. Coffee and tea both contain caffeine, a mild stimulant and diuretic, and the potassium content of coffee can be considerable. Fruit juices also provide potassium, and soft drinks contain much sugar and added phosphate. Alcohol provides 7 kcal per gram and some alcoholic beverages such as beer have a significant energy content which may contribute to obesity.

3.2 Dietary components

Most foods provide a spectrum of nutrients the availability of which will be influenced by the manner of preparation. Essential nutrients include protein, carbohydrate, fat, vitamins, minerals and trace elements. Information about the nutritional content of individual food items is beyond the scope of this book and should be sought in McCance and Widdowson (see the list of recommended reading).

3.2.1 PROTEIN

Protein contains nitrogen, sulphate, phosphate and carbohydrate. It is made up of chains of amino acids (see Fig. 2.6) which are linked by peptide bonds. Of the 20 amino acids found in man nine cannot be synthesized and must be supplied. These are known as essential amino acids, and are listed in Table 3.3. High-quality proteins such as meat and egg are rich in these amino acids.

3.2.2 CARBOHYDRATE

Dietary carbohydrate may be ingested in several forms.

Table 3.3 Essential amino acids

Histidine
Isoleucine
Leucine
Lysine
Methionine
Phenylalanine
Threonine
Tryptophan
Valine

(a) Monosaccharides

These are simple sugars of up to six carbon atoms which include trioses, tetroses, pentoses and hexoses. Examples of hexoses include glucose, fructose, galactose and mannose.

(b) Disaccharides

Lactose which consists of galactose and glucose is the most important disaccharide, and is the carbohydrate energy source in milk. Sucrose (fructose plus glucose) is a major component of the Western diet.

(c) Polysaccharides

Polysaccharides are polymers of glucose. They occur in two forms, starch and glycogen. Plants store carbohydrate as starch which is found in the form of amylose with alpha 1–4 links and amylopectin with alpha 1–4 and alpha 1–6 cross-links. The animal equivalent of starch is glycogen, which is discussed in Section 2.1.5.

(d) Fibre

Fibre is the skeletal remains of plant cells which are resistant to digestion by human enzymes. It includes cellulose and lignin. The importance of these dietary components has only recently been appreciated. Fibre is discussed further in Section 3.5.6 and fibre deficiency in relation to disease is reviewed in Chapter 7.

3.2.3 FATS

The majority of ingested fat is in the form of triglycerides, esters of glycerol and fatty acids (Fig. 2.1). Fatty acids of animal origin are saturated as are those derived from coconut palm kernel and cashew nuts. Unsaturated fatty acids which have one or more double bonds are found in vegetable oils, for example corn oil from maize. Vegetable oils are used increasingly in cooking and for the production of margarine. The clinical significance of saturated and polyunsaturated fats is discussed in Chapter 7. Other dietary fats include phospholipids and sterols such as cholesterol. The latter is found in high concentration in eggs and dairy produce.

3.2.4 VITAMINS

These are essential micronutrients. The metabolic role played by various vitamins is summarized in Section 2.4.5, and the clinical syndromes associated with vitamin deficiency are reviewed in Chapter 4. Important dietary sources of vitamins are listed in Table 3.4.

Table 3.4 Summary of some important dietary sources of vitamins

Vitamin	Important food sources
Vitamin A	Carrots Green leaf vegetables
Thiamin	Wholewheat Pulses Meat
Riboflavin	Liver Kidney Dairy produce
Niacin	Liver Kidney
Vitamin B6	Liver Whole grain cereals Nuts
Vitamin B12	Liver Meat Eggs Cheese
Folate	Liver Spinach Broccoli Cabbage
Vitamin C	Fruit Cabbage Potatoes
Vitamin D	Oily fish Fortified margarine Eggs
Vitamin E	Vegetable oils Margarine Eggs Butter
Vitamin K	Green vegetables Liver

(a) Vitamin A

Preformed Vitamin A is obtained from liver and fish oils as well as dairy products, eggs and fortified margarine. Beta carotene, which is supplied by carrots and green leaf vegetables such as broccoli and spinach, is cleaved by intestinal enzymes producing two molecules of Vitamin A. Storage is in the liver.

(b) Thiamin

Thiamin is widely distributed and much is obtained from cereals including wholewheat and fortified breakfast cereals. It is also present in meat. Nevertheless body stores are limited to approximately one month's supply and for this reason thiamin deficiency is not uncommon in hospital practice.

(c) Riboflavin

Riboflavin is available in a range of food products, particularly in liver, dairy produce and wheat bran. Much is obtained from fortified breakfast cereals.

(d) Niacin

Sources of niacin include meats, especially liver and kidney, pulses, nuts and wholewheat.

(e) Vitamin B6

In addition to pyridoxine Vitamin B6 refers to the related substances pyridoxal, pyridoxamine, and their 5-phosphate derivatives. Because it is widely distributed deficiency is uncommon, although as discussed in Chapter 9 some drugs may interreact with Vitamin B6.

(f) Vitamin B12

This is ingested in liver, meats and dairy produce. Large reserves are stored in the adult, dietary insufficiency is rare and is only found in the vegan. Deficiency when it occurs usually reflects absorptive defects as discussed in Chapter 2.

(g) Folate

Folate is present in liver, green vegetables and legumes, but the amount of vitamin supplied to the patient may be considerably reduced by inappropriate preparation such as over-cooking.

(h) Vitamin C

Vitamin C is also destroyed by over-cooking as well as by exposure to light. The main sources are citrus fruits and fresh green vegetables.

(i) Vitamin D

Exposure to sunlight leads to the production of cholecalciferol from 7 dehydrocholesterol in the skin. In many countries this is inadequate because of climate, pollution or social custom. Preformed Vitamin D is obtained from oily fish, eggs, fortified margarine and liver.

(j) Vitamin E

The richest source of Vitamin E is vegetable oils and margarine, but some is also obtained from eggs and butter.

(k) Vitamin K

Vitamin K_1 is largely derived from vegetables, and Vitamin K_2 is produced by intestinal bacteria.

3.2.5 MINERALS

(a) Calcium and phosphate

Dietary calcium is mostly obtained from dairy products such as milk and cheese. Root vegetables contribute significant amounts but there is very little calcium in potatoes. Phosphate is similarly obtained from dairy products and also from meat.

(b) Magnesium

Most foods contain magnesium. Foods of vegetable origin are a particularly important source because magnesium is an essential component of chlorophyll.

(c) Potassium

The potassium content of selected foods is shown in Table 3.5. Foods that are rich in potassium include chips, dried fruit and spinach as well as beverages such as coffee and orange juice. The consumption of these items needs to be limited in patients with renal failure.

(d) Sodium

The sodium content of some foods is shown in Table 3.6. The higher sodium content of processed foods is apparent and some convenience foods such as 'Chinese takeaway' have a very high content of mono-

Table 3.5 Potassium content of selected foods

Food	Potassium mmol/100 g
(a) *Foods with high potassium content*	
Potatoes	
Chips	26.9
Crisps	30.9
Roast	19.5
Baked	17.7
Cereals	
All-Bran	27.8
Muesli	15.6
Fruit	
Dried apricots	48.9
Banana	9.1
Stewed prunes	11.4
(b) *Foods with low potassium content*	
Boiled spaghetti	1.3
Boiled rice	1.0
Cornflakes	2.6
White bread	2.6
Sponge cake	2.1
Cottage cheese	1.4
Poached egg	2.9

Table 3.6 The sodium content of some foods (mmol/100 g)

Unprocessed food		Processed food	
Wholemeal flour	0.1	White bread	11
Beef	2.5	Beef sausages	35
Milk	2.3	Cheese	28
Boiled potatoes	1.8	Powdered potatoes	11

(Adapted from *Human Nutrition and Dietetics*, Passmore and Eastwood (eds), , Churchill Livingstone, 1986.)

sodium glutamate. Up to one third of dietary salt is added during cooking.

3.2.6 TRACE ELEMENTS

The essential trace elements are listed in Table 3.7. Food may also contain some elements such as barium and rubidium which serve no known function as well as elements such as lead and mercury which are potentially toxic. These will not be discussed further.

Table 3.7 Essential trace elements

*Iron	*Iodide
*Zinc	*Cobalt
*Manganese	Molybdenum
*Fluoride	Nickel
*Copper	Silicon
*Chromium	Tin
*Selenium	Vanadium

*Known to be clinically significant in man

(a) Iron

Whereas iron is widely available considerable variation in the iron content of foods is caused by different soil concentrations. Foods rich in iron include liver, beef, plain chocolate and some pulses. There is relatively little iron in milk so the baby is dependent on stores for the first few months. Hence prematurity or a delayed introduction of solid food leads to iron deficiency.

(b) Zinc

Zinc occurs in meat, fish, wholegrain cereals and legumes. However the availability in cereals may be reduced because of binding to phytate. This problem is circumvented by fermentation with yeast which degrades the phytate.

(c) Miscellaneous trace elements

Sources of manganese include unrefined grain, vegetables, nuts and fruit. Fluoride is mainly obtained from drinking water. Copper is principally ingested in liver, shellfish, nuts and wheat. Foods rich in chromium include liver, meat, cheese and wholewheat. Meat and seafood provide most selenium and cobalt. Iodide is mainly obtained from seafood.

3.3 Food additives

A variety of additives is employed during the commercial preparation of food to preserve, stabilize or enhance the product. There are more than one thousand additives some of which may have important clinical implications which are discussed in Chapter 8. Some are natural products. Examples of common food additives are listed in Table 3.8.

Preservatives are used in regulated concentrations in certain foods. Examples include sulphur dioxide in dried fruit and nitrates in bacon and ham. Antioxidants including propyl gallate and tocopherols retard oxidation and thus delay rancidity in oils and fats.

The colour of food may be enhanced by natural additives such as beetroot red or beta carotene, or by synthetic colours like tartrazine. Food texture can be modified with thickening agents like pectin, guar gum or carboxymethyl cellulose. Fat extending agents stabilize fat emulsions and allow the addition of more water, for example during the manufacture of ice cream. Chemicals are also used to modify

Table 3.8 Examples of common food additives

Purpose	Additive	Code
Preservatives	Benzoic acid	E 210
	Sodium metabisulphate	E 223
Antioxidants	Propyl gallate	E 310
	Tocopherols	E 306–9
Emulsifiers	Lecithins	E 322
	Monoglycerides	E 471
Thickeners	Guar gum	E 412
	Carboxymethyl cellulose	E 466
Colours	Chlorophyll	E 140
	Tartrazine	E 102

(Adapted from Truswell, A. S. and Brand, J. C. (1985) Processing Food, *British Medical Journal*, 1186–1190.)

flavour. There are sweetening compounds like saccharin, and monosodium glutamate is alleged to provide a meaty taste when added to soups and stews.

With the exception of flavourings all additives must now be identified by serial numbers on each food item. Foods are also monitored under the auspices of the UK Ministry of Agriculture for unintentional contamination by farm or industrial chemicals including fertilizers, pesticides and plasticizers.

3.4 Food processing

Food processing fulfils several functions. It improves the palatability, quality and safety of food while facilitating storage and convenience of presentation. Not all processes can achieve these objectives and compromises are inevitable.

3.4.1 MILLING

Cereals are milled to remove the outer layers and enhance their palatability. Low extraction flours are those from which a relatively high proportion of the cereal has been discarded as bran. Because of the uneven distribution of nutrients within wheat there are large losses of water soluble vitamins such as thiamin and nicotinic acid as well as calcium, zinc and fibre from such flours. Consequently in Britain and the USA these flours are fortified with additives such as water soluble vitamins, Vitamin D and minerals such as calcium and iron.

Fortification does not occur in underdeveloped countries where the development of new milling techniques has compounded the effect of poor diet by significantly reducing the nutritive value of cereals. Thus the thiamin content of husked rice of $4 \mu g/g$ can be reduced to $0.7 \mu g/g$ by the time it is polished.

3.4.2 PASTEURIZATION AND STERILIZATION

This is a process in which food such as milk is heated for short periods either to reduce the population of micro-organisms (pasteurization) or to eliminate micro-organisms entirely (sterilization). The temperature and duration of heating will determine the microbiological outcome as well as the influence on flavour.

Pasteurization eliminates important gastrointestinal pathogens such as Salmonella and Campylobacter species. These are common causes of gastroenteritis and community outbreaks have followed a breakdown of the pasteurization process. The subject of food infection is discussed in Chapter 8. Sterilization greatly prolongs shelf life but the higher temperatures involved have a greater impact on flavour. Both processes involve loss of Vitamin C but this is inconsequential as milk is an unimportant source of this vitamin.

3.4.3 IRRADIATION

Gamma irradiation is likely to be used increasingly for food sterilization as a convenient alternative to heat. It is commonly used to sterilize food for immunocompromised patients. There is relatively little effect on food composition although vitamin losses occur in some foods: this particularly applies to thiamin.

3.4.4 BLANCHING

Food is heated for brief periods to inactivate enzymes that would otherwise cause deterioration after freezing. This and the subsequent water cooling leads to loss of some vitamins and minerals.

3.4.5 FREEZING

Freezing is the best method of food storage and involves relatively little nutrient loss. Most losses occur during blanching and after thawing.

3.4.6 CANNING

Canned foods have to be sterilized and this process may cause nutritional losses. Storage is associated with a reduction in Vitamin A and Vitamin E and a small reduction in protein quality. Other vitamins such as riboflavin, pyridoxine and folate are well preserved.

3.4.7 COOKING

Cooking renders food digestible and palatable. It also ensures the elimination of bacterial pathogens which frequently contaminate uncooked meats especially poultry. Cooking is inevitably associated with nutrient losses. The vitamins which are most susceptible to destruction include Vitamin C and folate. The content of thiamin and Vitamin B6 is reduced to a lesser extent. Such losses may be minimized by the avoidance of over-cooking and prolonged warming of cooked foods. Less important is the Maillard reaction between reducing sugars and amino acids that occurs on the surface layers of meat and bread and which leads to the reduced availability of lysine.

3.5 Nutritional requirements

Recommended nutritional allowances are regularly published by the Department of Health and Social Security in Britain and by similar government agencies elsewhere. For a detailed account of this subject the reader is referred to these sources. Such recommendations apply to healthy individuals, and do not necessarily satisfy the requirements of the ill or malnourished hospital patient whose needs call for careful assessment.

3.5.1 ENERGY

Energy allowances relate to the needs of the healthy individual at rest. Adjustments have to be made for physical activity, body size, ambient temperature and age. Heavy labour requires the addition of up to 1500 kcal (6.29 MJ) per day. More energy is needed during pregnancy for foetal and placental development and an additional 120 kcal (0.5 MJ) per 100 ml of milk is recommended during lactation. Allowances are as high as 120 kcal (0.5 MJ) per kg after birth falling to 50 kcal (0.21 MJ) per kg by ten years of age. There is a 2% decline in resting metabolism for each decade in adults. Recommended amounts of food energy are shown in Tables 3.9 and 3.10.

3.5.2 PROTEIN

The minimum protein requirement based on measurements of obligatory nitrogen losses and nitrogen balance studies is shown in Table 3.11. These values refer to high-quality dairy protein. More protein will be needed when the diet is based on foods which contain low-quality protein with a lower essential amino acid content. Because the quantity of food eaten is largely determined by the energy content foods such as cassava and yams cannot be consumed in

Table 3.9 Recommended daily amounts of food energy in children

Age	Males		Females	
	kcal	MJ	kcal	MJ
1	1200	5.0	1100	4.5
2	1400	5.75	1300	5.5
3–4	1560	6.5	1500	6.25
5–6	1740	7.25	1680	7.0
7–8	1980	8.25	1900	8.0
9–11	2280	9.5	2050	8.5
12–14	2640	11.0	2150	9.0
15–17	2880	12.0	2150	9.0

(Adapted from D.H.S.S. *Report on Health and Social Subjects 15* (1979))

Table 3.10 Recommended daily amounts of food energy in adults

Age		Category	Energy	
			kcal	MJ
Men	18–34	Sedentary	2510	10.5
		Moderately active	2900	12.0
		Very active	3350	14.0
	35–64	Sedentary	2400	10.0
		Moderately active	2750	11.5
		Very active	3350	14.0
Women	18–54	Most occupations	2150	9.0
		Very active	2500	10.5
	55–74	Sedentary	1900	8.0

(Adapted from D.H.S.S. *Report on Health and Social Subjects 15* (1979))

sufficient amounts to meet the protein requirements. Furthermore, the absorption of amino acids from protein of vegetable origin may be less complete than that from protein of animal sources.

Nine of the 20 amino acids present in human tissues cannot be synthesized. These nine essential amino acids are listed in Table 3.12 in which their requirements are summarized. More than 40% of the amino acids in milk and eggs are from this group.

Table 3.11 Recommended daily amounts of protein (g)

Age	Male	Female
1	30	27
5–6	43	42
9–11	57	51
15–17	72	53
18–34	63–84	54–62
35–64	60–84	

(Adapted from D.H.S.S. *Report on Health and Social Subjects 15* (1979))

Table 3.12 Essential amino acid requirements (mg/kg/day)*

Amino acid	Infants	Adults
Histidine	28	
Isoleucine	70	10
Leucine	161	14
Lysine	103	12
Methylamine and cystine	58	13
Phenylalanine and tyrosine	125	14
Threonine	87	7
Tryptophan	17	4
Valine	93	10

*(Modified from McLaren, D. S. (1980) *Nutrition and its Disorders*, 3rd edn, Churchill Livingstone, Edinburgh.)

3.5.3 VITAMINS

The daily vitamin needs of a healthy adult are shown in Table 3.13. It must be remembered that thiamin requirements are dependent upon dietary carbohydrate. A high carbohydrate diet will increase the demands for thiamin. For this reason dextrose solutions are capable of precipitating Wernicke's encephalopathy in malnourished alcoholics, so thiamin supplements should be administered first. The requirement for folate is doubled in pregnancy and more Vitamin D is needed during growth and development. Additional vitamins should be provided in patients who are receiving total parenteral nutrition and renal dialysis. These subjects are discussed in Chapters 6 and 7.

Table 3.13 The daily vitamin requirements
in healthy adults

Vitamin A	1 mg
Thiamin	1.2 mg
Riboflavin	1.6 mg
Niacin	18 mg
Vitamin B6	3 mg
Vitamin B12	2 μg
Folate	200 μg
Vitamin C	30 mg
Vitamin D	3 μg
Vitamin E	10 mg
Vitamin K	100 μg

3.5.4 MINERALS

(a) Calcium

The recommended adult allowance is 500–700 mg per day. Whereas the greater needs during pregnancy and lactation are partially offset by enhanced intestinal absorption, intake should be increased to 1000–1300 mg per day under these circumstances.

(b) Iron

The recommended daily allowance for male subjects is 10 mg. The demands of menstruation and pregnancy call for increased dietary iron in females. During the childbearing years it was traditionally recommended that they should receive 12 mg daily increasing to 15 mg daily during lactation. Currently these estimates are considered to be low. Deficient iron stores or iron deficiency anaemia are commonly found in menstruating females. More recent recommendations suggest the need for 18 mg of iron a day in these female subjects.

(c) Miscellaneous trace elements

Various trace elements form an obligatory part of the diet as discussed in Section 3.2.6. These substances are widely distributed in food products and deficiency is very unlikely to occur except in those few

Table 3.14 Recommended intakes of trace
elements

Element	Intake (mg per day)
Zinc	15
Iodide	0.15
Manganese	2.5–5.0
Copper	2.0–3.0
Chromium	0.05–0.2
Selenium	0.05–0.2

patients who are receiving prolonged total parenteral nutrition. Recommended intakes of trace elements are listed in Table 3.14.

3.5.5 WATER AND ELECTROLYTE REQUIREMENTS

The normal adult will drink approximately 1.5–2 litres of water a day. This usually covers obligatory losses and facilitates production of sufficient urine to excrete waste products. The requirements for water and electrolytes vary considerably, particularly in ill patients. This subject is discussed in detail in Section 2.8.

3.5.6 FIBRE

For many years fibre was considered to have no nutritional significance. The reduced availability of calcium and zinc in the presence of some forms of dietary fibre was then recognized. More recently the increasing refinement of carbohydrate food with the exclusion of fibre has been incriminated in the genesis of a range of disorders including dental caries, obesity, cardiovascular disease and diseases of the intestine. Fibre influences satiety and intestinal pressures, and may bind chemicals such as degraded bile acids. The relationship of dietary fibre to disease is discussed in Chapter 7. In spite of an increasing awareness of the importance of dietary fibre consumption frequently falls short of the recommended daily intake of 25–30 g.

3.5.7 FAT

Fat is an expedient energy source with high energy density which contains essential fatty acids as well as some fat soluble vitamins. It is widely available and in the UK up to 40% of the total energy intake is provided by fat. The requirement for essential fatty acids is minimal and only in patients with the most severe protracted steatorrhoea or prolonged total parenteral nutrition will essential fatty acid deficiency arise. The problem is nearly always due to over-provision with the attendant risks of obesity and vascular disease which are discussed in Chapter 7.

3.6 The healthy diet

3.6.1 DIETARY PERSPECTIVE

The importance of diet in relation to obesity and the development of diseases of the cardiovascular, renal and gastrointestinal systems is gaining increasing recognition. This subject is discussed in more detail in Chapters 7 and 8. There is now a general appreciation that the typical British diet, as well as that eaten in many parts of Western Europe and the USA, requires modification.

In the British population one third of adults and 50% of subjects between the ages of 60 and 65 years are overweight, and a similar problem exists in the USA. There is therefore a need for the consumption of less energy-dense food. Such a change can be achieved partly by reducing the proportion of dietary fat and increasing the energy contribution from carbohydrate, and partly by increasing the proportion of unrefined carbohydrate and reducing the consumption of sugar. Much sugar is taken in the form of soft drinks and confectionery. Such changes would automatically lead to an increase in the consumption of fibre with additional beneficial effects, particularly in relation to disease of the gastrointestinal system.

The reduction in the consumption of dietary fat would help reduce cardiovascular morbidity, particularly if in addition the ratio of polyunsaturated to saturated fatty acids was increased. Furthermore the 'Western' diet has a high salt content, reduction of which may favourably influence the incidence of hypertension. This is readily achieved by avoiding salt-rich processed foods and by reducing the amount of salt which is added to food during cooking.

3.6.2 DIETARY GOALS

The ideal diet is an unrealistic concept but on the basis of currently available information various authorities, including the World Health

Table 3.15   Summary of some of the NACNE recommendations

Dietary component	Current intake	NACNE recommendations	
		Short-term	Long-term
Total fat	38% of total energy	34% of total energy	30% of total energy
Saturated fat	18% of total energy	15% of total energy	10% of total energy
Sugar	38 kg per year	34 kg per year	20 kg per year
Fibre	20 g per day	25 g per day	30 g per day

Organization, have recommended desirable dietary objectives which are designed to improve national health. The nature of the requisite changes will depend upon the characteristics of the national diet and the disease pattern in the country under consideration. Similar dietary modifications are required in Britain and the USA, and these are also applicable to countries where the 'Western' diet has been adopted. Major dietary changes are unlikely to be achieved abruptly, and recommendations must be based on measures that are practical and acceptable as outlined in Britain by the National Advisory Committee on Nutrition Education (NACNE 1983). These recommendations are summarized in Table 3.15. Introduction of the short-term proposals is envisaged during the 1980s and adoption of long-term proposals is anticipated over the next 15 years. The recommendations may be summarized as follows.

(a) Fat

A reduction in the food energy obtained from fat from 38% to 34% of the total calories, with a reduction in the saturated fat from 18% to 15% of the total energy content. Corresponding recommendations from the World Health Organization suggest that currently no more than 30% of energy should be derived from fat and 10% from saturated fats. The latter may be applicable to specific patients but can lead to problems of dietary palatability and compliance.

(b) Carbohydrate

There should be a reduction in the food energy obtained from sugar from 14% to 12%. Some authorities have suggested that sugar consumption be reduced by half. The overall food energy obtained from carbohydrate should be increased to 50% of the total with a substantial increase in the amount of fibre. The average British diet contains 20 g of fibre a day, and an immediate increase to 25 g a day is recommended but 30–50 g may be preferable. People in the Third World eat up to 150 g of fibre per day but such large intakes reduce mineral absorption and may lead to energy deprivation in children.

(c) Miscellaneous recommendations

A reduction in the present level of daily salt consumption of 7–12 g is recommended, and alcohol should account for no more than 5% of the total energy intake.

3.6.3 IMPLEMENTATION OF THE NUTRITIONAL GUIDELINES

The recommended dietary improvements can be achieved by simple modification of the national diet. The desirable changes may be achieved as follows.

(a) Fat

The total fat consumption may be reduced by grilling rather than frying food, the use of skimmed or semi-skimmed milk and by avoiding the excessive consumption of dairy products such as eggs, cream and high-fat cheese. The use of margarine containing poly-unsaturates and vegetable oil for cooking will further reduce saturated fat consumption.

(b) Carbohydrate

The use of high fibre cereals, wholewheat bread and increased consumption of fruit and vegetables will raise the intake of carbohydrates and fibre. Sugar consumption is reduced by the use of sugar substitutes and by eating less sweets and confectionery.

(c) Salt

Half of the salt consumed is added during or after cooking and a significant amount of salt is ingested in processed foods (e.g. crisps,

Chinese takeaways). Consequently there is considerable scope for the reduction of dietary salt.

Dietary habits are influenced by many factors. The increasing dependence on convenience foods, which are frequently rich in energy, fats, salt and additives with little fibre, is partly due to an increase in the proportion of women who are in paid employment. Many of the traditional domestic skills have been lost and during a recession there are financial pressures from a dwindling domestic budget to limit expenditure on food. The mistaken belief that food of better nutritional quality is necessarily more expensive is prevalent.

Significant improvements in diet can only be achieved through education. There is evidence that eating habits are worse in social classes IV and V and that the housewife principally determines the family diet. Dietary education begins in the school curriculum and is reinforced by health care professionals at antenatal and well baby clinics and during contact with ill patients. Increasingly hospital and school catering departments are offering more appropriate menus. The quality of processed food is being improved with the co-operation of manufacturers. This has led to a reduction of the salt content of many items and the wide availability of semi-skimmed milk.

3.7 Nutrition in childhood, pregnancy and old age

3.7.1 NUTRITION IN INFANTS, CHILDREN AND ADOLESCENTS

During the first six months of life energy requirements are 115 kcal/kg (0.48 MJ). Basal requirements are high at 55 kcal/kg (0.23 MJ) because of heat loss due to the relatively large surface area. Thirty-five kcal/kg (0.15 MJ) are required for growth and 10–25 kcal/kg (0.04–0.1 MJ) for activity. The corresponding protein requirement is 2.2 g/kg. In the second six months the infant needs 105 kcal and 2 g of protein/kg. These needs are ideally met with breast milk. This provides 79 kcal/100 ml (0.33 MJ), 7% from protein, 55% from fat and 38% from carbohydrate. The carbohydrate is in the form of lactose which supplies galactose, a necessary component of myelin in nerve fibres and collagen in connective tissue, and the fat is rich in linoleic acid.

A child's diet is mainly governed by the mother. Nutrition may be adversely influenced by the excessive consumption of sugar in the form of sweets and confectionery: these represent empty calories which lack other nutrients, contribute to dental caries and, when taken between meals, depress the appetite at meal-times and thus impair the consumption of a more satisfactory diet. Food fads should be discouraged, and the child should eat from each of the basic food groups every day which collectively include all the essential nutrients.

The adolescent growth spurt of up to 10 cm and 5 kg in one year imposes large nutritional demands. It frequently occurs at the age of 12 years in girls and 14 years in boys. During this time the child may consume up to 4000 kcal (16.8 MJ) per day. Conversely some adolescents begin to diet at this stage, a few may be overweight but others wish to conform to a thin model image.

Specific nutrient deficiencies may include iron and calcium. Inadequate stores of Vitamin A, Vitamin C and zinc have also been demonstrated in some studies. Iron deficiency is common in adolescent females who are growing, menstruating and restricting their diet. During the peak growth velocity, the accretion of calcium into the skeleton may reach 100 g per year, and because dietary absorption is 20%, 1400 mg of calcium may be needed each day. This can readily be provided by encouraging the consumption of milk and preferably by substituting milk for sugar-laden soft drinks.

3.7.2 NUTRITION DURING PREGNANCY AND LACTATION

(a) Pregnancy

Pregnancy is accompanied by a weight gain of 11–12.5 kg. Weight increases by 1–2 kg during the first trimester and thereafter by 400 g a week until term. Approximately 5 kg of this increase is accounted for by maternal stores which include 4 kg of fat.

The pregnant woman requires an additional energy consumption 300 kcal per day (1.5 MJ) and the equivalent of an additional 10 g of high-quality protein. Calcium and phosphorus intake should both be increased by 400 mg per day and thus the recommended daily calcium intake is 1200 mg, equivalent to one litre of milk. Interest is currently focused on zinc, but whereas some pregnant women appear deficient in zinc, and deficiency correlates with small-for-dates foetuses, more information is required before firm guidelines can be issued. Many women have low or absent iron stores and iron supplements are usually supplied to meet the increased demands. Folate requirements are doubled and without supplements one third of pregnant women would be in negative balance in both Britain and the USA. Because low folate concentrations correlate with a poor outcome of pregnancy, and possibly neural tube defects early in pregnancy, folate supplements are usually prescribed. The need for other water soluble and fat soluble vitamins is increased, especially for Vitamin D.

These requirements emphasize the importance of dietetic counselling in early pregnancy, or even before conception. When such a service is available routine haematinic and vitamin supplements can be omitted in the majority of patients.

(b) Lactation

Human milk provides 70 kcal per 100 ml, the production of which requires 90 kcal. Consequently the daily energy availability of 800 kcal (3.4 MJ) is needed for the average daily production of 850 ml of milk. Assuming that the 4 kg of fat laid down during the pregnancy is available for milk production the recommended additional daily energy allowance during lactation is 500 kcal (2.1 MJ). This value may need to be increased if feeding continues beyond three months. It will also need to be modified according to the volume of milk produced and the mother's weight.

The additional needs of the lactating mother are best met with milk and an increase in the consumption of meat, citrus fruits and vegetables. If the mother does not like milk, calcium supplements will be required to meet the recommended daily allowance of 1200 mg.

3.7.3 NUTRITION IN OLD AGE

There is a growing elderly population in this country as in many other Western societies. Recent attention has been focused on the problem of malnutrition that exists in a significant proportion of elderly subjects.

A reduction in muscle mass occurs after the age of 40 years and with this there is a reduction in the basal metabolic rate by 2% each decade. Thus energy requirements are less in the elderly than in the young (see Table 3.10). Nevertheless inadequate intake of macronutrients and micronutrients frequently occurs in this population for the reasons

Table 3.16   Factors associated with dietary
inadequacy in the elderly

Social isolation
Economic hardship
Depression
Concomitant disease
Drug therapy

listed in Table 3.16. People who live alone may not bother to prepare
meals. Many elderly patients have limited financial resources and are
too proud to accept state benefits to which they are entitled.
Depression may be a feature of social isolation as well as a result of
concomitant disease. Disease may reduce their mobility and ability to
prepare food, for example rheumatoid arthritis, or impair the appetite
particularly in gastrointestinal disease and neoplasia, or require drug
therapy which may also lead to anorexia.

The provision of an adequate and well balanced-diet for this
population is an important contribution to the quality of life and
enhances their ability to contend with underlying disease.

References

Hanssen, M. (1984) *E for Additives*, Thorsons, Wellingborough.

National Advisory Committee on Nutritional Education (NACNE) (1983) *A
Discussion Paper on the Proposals for Nutritional Guidelines for Health
Education in Britain*, Health Education Council, London.

Passmore, R. and Eastwood, M. A. (1986) *Human Nutrition and Dietetics*, 8th
Edn, Churchill Livingstone, Edinburgh.

Paul, A. A. and Southgate, D. A. T. (1978) *McCance and Widdowson, The
Composition of Foods*, 4th Edn, HMSO, London.

Royal College of Physicians (1981) *Report on Medical Aspects of Dietary Fibre*,
HMSO, London.

W.H.O. Technical report series (1982) *Prevention of coronary heart disease*, **678**,
5–53.

4

MALNUTRITION

Inadequate, excessive or inappropriate nutrition is a universal phenomenon. Medical problems arise as a consequence of both under-nutrition and over-nutrition. This chapter is primarily concerned with the recognition, consequences and causes of under-nutrition. Diseases associated with excessive food intake are discussed in more detail in Chapter 7.

Traditional medical attention has focused on the pathogenesis, recognition and management of disease, and the problem of associated malnutrition has been ignored. Macronutrient deficiency, such as protein and energy malnutrition, was regarded as a Third World affliction and nutritional interest in hospital practice was until recently restricted to specific micronutrient deficiencies occurring in the context of specific disease. Examples of the latter include haematinic deficiency in gluten enteropathy, Vitamin B12 deficiency in pernicious anaemia, and zinc deficiency in dermatitis enteropathica. The recognition that almost half of all patients in acute hospitals are under-nourished and suffer from macronutrient deficiency has been a relatively recent development. Nutritional deficiencies occur most commonly in surgical practice, and this problem is exacerbated by the decline in nutritional status of surgical patients during the period of hospital stay. Medical patients are also affected, particularly those with cancer, alcoholic liver disease and chronic respiratory disease. Conversely many of the features of gross malnutrition in the Third World are not entirely attributable to macronutrient deficiency and it has become clear that micronutrients such as trace elements have great importance. The difference between marasmus with wasting and stunting and kwashiorkor with the additional features of oedema, dermatitis, discoloured hair and hepatomegaly, may not simply reflect the relative protein deficiency of the latter but a depletion of chormium, selenium and manganese. Hence malnutrition is a common problem in which both macronutrients and micronutrients are of importance. The problem of clinical malnutrition in hospital practice has attracted recent attention and interest for a variety of reasons. These may be summarized as follows:

- The recognition that malnutrition is common in hospital practice has been accompanied by an appreciation of the morbidity and mortality that is associated with nutritional impairment
- The development of intensive care has led to an increase in the number of patients with multi-system failure who require nutritional support as part of their management
- There has been an increase in the incidence of Crohn's disease which is an important cause of under-nutrition and intestinal failure
- There is an ageing population with an increased prevalence of chronic disease associated with nutritional deficiency

4.1 The recognition of malnutrition

The majority of malnourished patients have deficiencies of many nutrients. Each deficiency may be associated with one or more biochemical abnormalities which can ultimately lead to disordered physiology and structural change. Consequently no single clinical or laboratory marker will satisfactorily assess nutritional status. Current methods of nutritional assessment are individually inadequate but collectively useful. Many are applied not only for the recognition of malnutrition but for patient monitoring during nutritional support. In spite of an array of clinical, anthropometric and laboratory parameters which are employed for this purpose, clinical judgement by an experienced observer is equally affective in the identification of patients with significant nutritional depletion.

4.1.1 CLINICAL ASSESSMENT

(a) Primary disease

Most patients exhibit clinical features of the disease responsible for malnutrition. Examples include abdominal pain and diarrhoea associated with Crohn's disease, the peripheral neuropathy or hepatic disease of alcohol abuse, the respiratory symptoms associated with bronchial carcinoma, and psychomotor retardation of depression. Such features should prompt consideration of nutritional status.

(b) Diet

A dietary history is often confined to dietary recall. This relies on memory which is frequently fallible and may relate to an unrepresentative day. Undoubtedly the most accurate method of dietary assessment involves a prospective food intake record in which individual foods are itemized and preferably weighed. Unfortunately this is a major undertaking which is unacceptable to many patients. Much useful information may be derived from simple questions about the number and nature of meals, likes and dislikes, and simple snacks. This provides an adequate indication of protein and energy intake as well as highlighting potential deficiencies. These include Vitamin C and folate in patients who do not consume sufficient fruit or vegetables.

(c) Symptoms and signs

Significient protein energy malnutrition is accompanied by inertia and lethargy which may be misinterpreted by the inexperienced clinician as depression or unco-operative behaviour. Deficiency of specific nutrients produces clinical features but generally these lack sensitivity and specificity and their absence does not necessarily indicate adequate nutrition. Specific syndromes of nutrient deficiency are discussed in Section 4.2.

Inspection of the skin will reveal loss of fat which is accompanied by wrinkling in the elderly and lanugo hair in the young. Reduction in muscle size may occur rapidly in the stressed patient particularly in the presence of sepsis. Nevertheless muscle wasting is frequently overlooked especially in the obese subject. Malnutrition is obvious when it is severe (Fig. 4.1). It should be recognized long before this stage is reached.

A dry flaky skin may be a feature of essential fatty acid deficiency, and pigmentation may imply niacin deficiency. Follicular hyperkeratosis is a rare feature which occurs in Vitamin A deficiency, and perifollicular haemorrhages are found in scorbutaemia in addition to bruising which also occurs with insufficient Vitamin K. Malnutrition

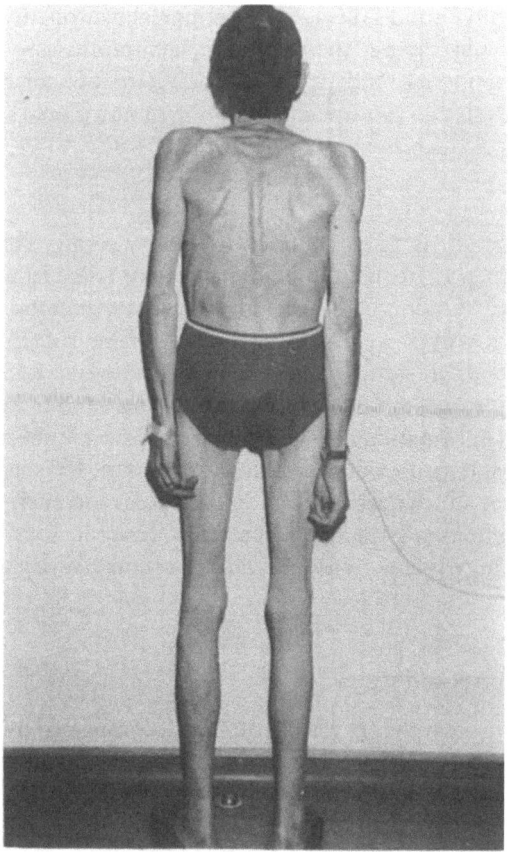

Figure 4.1 Patient with Crohn's disease, ankylosing spondylitis and
moderate to severe malnutrition

is accompanied by hair thinning, leukonykia and nail ridging, and
anaemia is common.

Cheilosis and angular stomatitis previously attracted much attention. Both may respond to Vitamin B replacement. Whereas angular
stomatitis is occasionally a feature of iron deficiency, it may simply be
a manifestation of deeper creases in edentulous patients. Glossitis
accompanies deficiency of the haematinics Vitamin B12, folate and
iron. Swollen ulcerated gums occurs in patients with Vitamin C
deficiency but not in the edentulous.

Abnormalities of the central nervous system are especially

important. Reference has already been made to the lethargy which follows protein energy malnutrition, and drowsiness or even coma can accompany hypophosphataemia. Complaints of diplopia, particularly if associated with nystagmus and ataxia prompt consideration of thiamin deficiency which can also be responsible for loss of short-term memory. Dementia has been attributed to niacin and Vitamin B12 deficiency, but the latter is more commonly associated with neurological damage affecting the spinal cord and peripheral nerves. Impaired tendon reflexes and extensor plantar responses are typical of the syndrome of sub-acute combined degeneration of the cord. Peripheral neuropathy or spinal disease may be caused by essential fatty acid deficiency. Finally skeletal deformity or bone tenderness is indicative of Vitamin D deficiency which also leads to proximal myopathy.

4.1.2 ANTHROPOMETRIC MEASUREMENTS

(a) Weight and height

The accurate measurement of weight is helpful but it must be remembered that rapid fluctuations reflect fluid balance rather than nutritional status. Patients should be weighed without clothing and at the same time each day. Height measurement is essential in young patients. Changes in growth velocity may indicate changes in nutritional status or disease activity. The patient is placed on a stadiometer without shoes or socks with the heels together, feet parallel and straight knees. The Frankfurt plane, the line between the lower border of the left orbit and the upper margin of the external auditory meatus, should be horizontal.

(b) Skin fold thickness

Skin fold thickness is used as a simple measure of body fat. This measurement is valueless in the obese and misleading in the oedematous. Minor differences in technique can lead to large differences in results, variation between observers masks small changes and consequently assessment by a single observer for monitoring purposes is recommended. Because of differences in fat distribution, for example fat is more centrally distributed in diabetics, it is customary to obtain the sum of measurements at four sites. These are

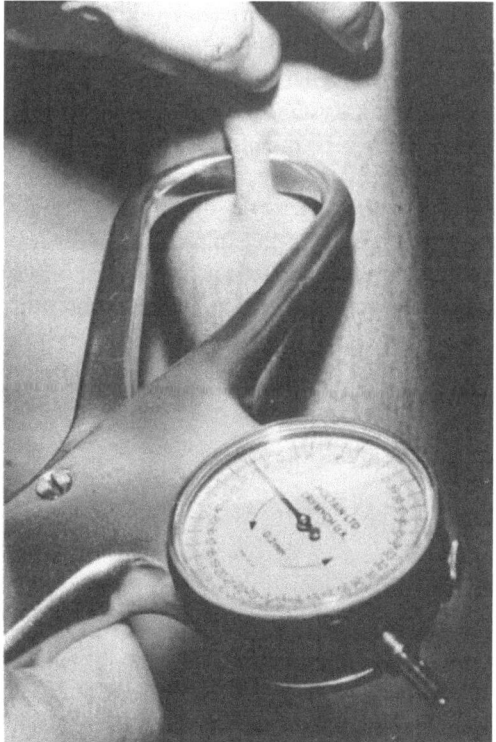

Figure 4.2 The measurement of triceps skin fold thickness

triceps, biceps, subscapular fold and iliac crest. When individual patients are being monitored the triceps thickness alone is sufficient.

Triceps skin fold thickness is measured posteriorly at the mid-point of the left arm. The patient stands with the left arm hanging freely and a mid-point is marked halfway between the lower border of the acromial process of the scapula and the tip of the olecranon process. A skin fold is held between the observer's finger and thumb 1 cm above the mid-point in line with the olecranon process (Fig. 4.2). Harpenden calipers are applied at the mid-point, the skin fold is released and a reading obtained after two seconds. The process is repeated three times and the mean of the two closest readings is recorded.

The biceps skin fold thickness is also measured at the mid-point in a similar fashion but with the subject sitting and the supinated forearm resting on the thigh. The subscapular fold is also measured on the left side with the subject sitting and is read at the lower scapular border with the calipers pointing downwards and laterally at 45°. Supra–iliac skin fold thickness is taken above the iliac crest in the mid-axillary line.

(c) Mid-arm circumference and mid-arm muscle circumference

This measurement is often used as a simple measure of body muscle. It is also influenced by oedema and variations in technique. The mid-arm circumference is obtained at the mid-point of the left arm and the mid-arm muscle circumference is derived from this and from the triceps skin fold thickness using the formula:

Muscle circumference = arm circumference (cm) − (π × tricep skin fold thickness (mm))

Adult standards for these anthropometric indices are given in Table 4.1.

(d) Dynometry

Recently it has become apparent that muscle function may be a more sensitive index of impaired nutrition than muscle size. This has led to the measurement of grip strength using a dynometer in the assessment

Table 4.1   Adult standards for anthropometric measurements

	Triceps skin fold thickness (mm)		
	Standard	80% of standard	60% of standard
Male	12.5	10.0	7.7
Female	16.5	13.2	9.9
	Arm muscle circumference (cm)		
	Standard	80% of standard	60% of standard
Male	25.3	20.2	15.2
Female	23.2	18.6	13.9

and monitoring of nutritional status. Although this technique has many advocates, results are subject to other factors than muscle strength, notably the patient's ability or willingness to co-operate.

(e) Body mass index

This is a simple index derived statistically from population data on weights and heights. It is measured by the formula:

$$\frac{Weight\ (kg)}{[Height\ (m)^2]}$$

Normal values for body mass index are discussed in Section 7.13. It is commonly used as an index of obesity, but it cannot distinguish between overweight due to excess fat or to muscle hypertrophy.

4.1.3 LABORATORY MEASUREMENTS

Nutritional assessment is facilitated by a wide range of laboratory measurements. Most of these are routinely available in every district general hospital.

(a) Electrolytes

Significant disturbance of water and electrolyte balance is a common feature in severe malnutrition particularly in patients who have trauma sepsis and multi-system disease. Abnormalities of sodium, potassium, water and acid-base status should always receive attention prior to the institution of nutritional support.

(b) Proteins

Serum albumin and transferrin provide evidence of visceral proteins status and low levels are restored by nutritional repletion. The rate of albumin synthesis is slow with a half life of 16–18 days; the half life of transferrin is 6–8 days. Whereas these measurements may represent useful indices particularly when recorded sequentially in the stable patient, interpretation is frequently difficult because of other factors which influence serum concentration. These include fluid shifts with haemodilution or haemoconcentration, impaired synthesis in liver disease and excessive loss through the renal or gastrointestinal tract.

Increased vascular permeability affects protein concentration significantly in the septic patient and iron deficiency tends to increase serum transferrin values as does the oral contaceptive. Recently the measurement of fibronectin has been advocated for nutritional assessment. This is an acute phase protein which is synthesized by the liver and facilitates phagocytosis. Whereas serum values fall and rise within three to five days in response to starvation and nutritional support, fibronectin concentrations are elevated in the presence of sepsis.

(c) Haematology

After correction of fluid and electrolyte imbalance a haemoglobin estimation may indicate anaemia. Inspection of the blood film may prompt the measurement of serum or red cell folate, Vitamin B12, iron and total iron binding capacity or transferrin. Prolongation of the prothrombin time is indicative of Vitamin K deficiency in the presence of normal liver function.

(d) Minerals and trace elements

The serum values of calcium, zinc, magnesium and iron are routinely obtained. However the measurement of trace elements such as selenium and chromium is more difficult and requires special methods of blood collection. This is normally a supra-regional service which is only required in patients who need prolonged total parenteral nutrition.

(e) Vitamins

Measurement of vitamins is also less widely available. Some of the methods employed are shown in Table 4.2

(f) Immunology

Immunological parameters are also used to monitor malnourished patients who have reduced lymphocyte counts and loss of delayed hypersensitivity reaction on skin testing. Unfortunately the latter lacks specificity, anergy being a common feature in many diseases associated with malnutrition, and these measurements are of doubtful value.

Table 4.2 Some laboratory methods used for the diagnosis of vitamin deficiency

Vitamin A	Plasma retinal
	Plasma carotene
Thiamin	RBC transketolase
	Urinary thiamin
Riboflavin	RBC glutathione reductase
	Urinary riboflavin
Pyridoxine	RBC glutamic oxaloacetic transaminase
	Urinary pyridoxic acid
Vitamin C	Leukocyte ascorbic acid
Vitamin D	Plasma 25 hydroxy cholecalciferol
Vitamin E	*In vitro* RBC haemolysis with H_2O_2
	Plasma tocopherol

(g) Nitrogen balance

Nitrogen balance studies are employed more frequently, usually for the purpose of monitoring nutritional support. Nitrogen from protein breakdown is largely converted to urea, thus the daily nitrogen loss may be estimated from the urea excreted in the urine with allowance being made for any change in blood urea concentration during this time. It may be conveniently calculated using the following formula:

Nitrogen loss (g) = mmol urinary urea per 24 h × 0.028 + 2

(2 approximates to the non-urinary nitrogen loss)

$\pm$ change in blood urea per 24 h (mmol) × 0.028 × $\dfrac{60}{100}$

× body weight (kg)

+ urinary protein loss (g) ÷ 6.25

Gastrointestinal losses are more difficult to predict.

(h) Miscellaneous measurements

The creatinine height index has been used as a measurement of lean body mass. It is believed that urinary creatinine excretion is related to the weight of skeletal muscle and correlation has been demonstrated between urinary creatinine, oxygen consumption and lean body mass. Reduction of body protein is associated with a reduction in creatinine excretion. Comparing the 24 hour urinary creatinine excretion by the patient with that expected by a normal individual of the same height and ideal weight provides information about nutritional status which is independent of fluid shifts. The creatinine height index is derived from the formula:

$$\frac{\text{measured urinary creatinine}}{\text{ideal urinary creatinine}} \times 100$$

Values for ideal creatinine are shown in Table 4.3. An index below 80% is abnormal and below 50% is indicative of severe muscle wasting. Unfortunately the usefulness of this index is reduced for various reasons. Creatinine excretion is reduced in renal failure, glycine and arginine are metabilized to creatinine and some nitrogen sources used in parenteral nutrition are rich in glycine. The measurement also involves assumptions about the patient's frame size.

Muscle breakdown releases 3 methyl histidine which is excreted unchanged in the urine. Measurement of urinary 3 methyl histidine has been used as a marker of muscle breakdown. Human adult muscle contains on average 4.2 μmol/g of protein. This estimation is difficult

Table 4.3 Values for 'ideal' urinary creatinine

	Men			Women	
Height (cm)	Ideal creatinine (mg)		Height (cm)	Ideal creatinine (mg)	
157.5	1288		147.3	830	
165.1	1386		154.9	900	
170.2	1467		160.0	949	
175.3	1555		165.1	1006	
180.3	1642		170.2	1076	
185.4	1739		175.3	1141	
190.5	1831		180.3	1206	

(From Blackburn, G. L., and Thornton, P. A. (1979) Symposium on Applied Nutrition in Clinical Practice. *Medical Clinics of North America*, 1095–1115.)

and is not widely used. Furthermore considerable doubt has been cast on the specificity of this measurement.

4.1.4 COMMON INDICES OF PROTEIN ENERGY MALNUTRITION

Some of the measurements which are commonly used as evidence of protein energy malnutrition are shown in Table 4.4. Each has to be interpreted in relation to the factors discussed previously, and trends are usually more meaningful than single readings. More detailed information about nutritional status may be obtained by the use of stable isotopes which provide important metabolic insight and will find increasing application in metabolic investigations. Such techniques are not currently available for routine clinical practice.

Table 4.4 Measurements commonly used for identifying protein energy malnutrition

Weight loss	>10%
Triceps skin fold thickness	<10 mm men
	<13 mm women
Arm muscle circumference	<23 cm men
	<22 cm women
Serum albumin	<35 g/l
Serum transferrin	<2 g/l
Lymphocyte count	<1500/μl

4.2 The consequences of malnutrition

Clinical disorders due to malnutrition can be conveniently considered in two groups, those due to macronutrient deficiency of protein and energy, and those caused by micronutrient deficency including vitamins and trace elements. However the fact that these deficiencies are usually combined merits emphasis. The requirements and metabolism of energy substrate, nitrogen, vitamins, and trace elements are considered in more detail in Chapters 2 and 3. Features resulting from nutrient deficiency are discussed here.

4.2.1 PROTEIN ENERGY MALNUTRITION

This problem is closely associated with the Third World, afflicting over one hundred million children over the age of five years and leading to the classical clinical spectrum of marasmus and kwashiorkor. The marasmic child has gross wasting of muscle and fat but is alert, hungry and free of oedema. Growth retardation and hypothermia may be evident in both marasmus and kwashiorkor conditions, but patients with kwashiorkor exhibit other features such as hypoalbuminaemic oedema, moon-shaped face, discoloured red hair, hepatomegaly and irritability. Body fat may be normal or increased. The original supposition that kwashiorkor represents protein deficiency is not supported by field studies. Other explanations for the two syndromes include different hormonal response, with high cortisol values occurring in patients with kwashiorkor, and differences in micronutrient status.

Protein energy malnutrition in hospital patients may also present with a spectrum of features. Patients who are otherwise well but who restrict their diet, such as those with anorexia nervosa, develop the features of marasmus. They become wasted but the serum albumin concentration is maintained. Conversely patients who are stressed with sepsis may appear less wasted but rapidly develop hypoalbuminaemic oedema and become apathetic and withdrawn. Major complications arise as a consequence. Immunity is impaired, there is a reduction of muscle function and thus respiratory function, and wound healing is delayed. Immobility contributes to the development of respiratory infection and wound infection also occurs more frequently. Infection imposes nutritional demands on the depleted patient.

Protein energy malnutrition is thus associated with increased mortality. However it is important to emphasize that whereas muscle wasting in malnourished stressed hospital patients is a feature of depressed muscle protein synthesis and possibly enhanced protein metabolism in visceral tissue, malnutrition is only one factor in their pathogenesis. Furthermore in spite of the widespread use of nutritional support amounting to a financial investment of millions of pounds, there is little evidence that intensive nutritional support reverses the wasting of cancer sepsis and chronic disease without management of the underlying disorder.

4.2.2 DEFICIENCY OF MICRONUTRIENTS

(a) Vitamins

Vitamin deficiency syndromes are common in the Third World but still occur in developed countries. Deficiencies of thiamin, folate, Vitamin C and Vitamin D are not rare in the United Kingdom where they are frequently overlooked. The causes of deficiency syndromes will be discussed in Section 4.3.

(i) Vitamin A   Vitamin A deficiency has a major impact on the eye. Defective dark adaption leads ultimately to night blindness. Impairment of mucus secreting epithelia causes xerophthalmia and corneal damage may lead to the loss of vision. The role of Vitamin A in the protection against epithelial cancer is uncertain, but the maintenance of the integrity of the epithelium is an important protective factor against infection. It must also be remembered that excessive Vitamin A is toxic leading acutely to headache, drowsiness and skin desquamation, and with chronic administration to weakness, bone hyperosteosis and liver damage.

(ii) Thiamin   Thiamin deficiency may readily develop in hospital practice because of limited body stores which amount to a month's provision. The nervous and cardiovascular systems are principally affected.

Neurological damage may take two forms. Ophthalmoplegia, nystagmus, ataxia, and mental confusion herald the Wernicke-Korsakoff syndrome which if untreated will lead to irreversible short-term memory impairment. Polyneuropathy (dry beriberi) presents with paraesthesia, cramps and impaired sensation. Cardiovascular beriberi is characterized by biventricular cardiac failure, dyspnoea and oedema.

(iii) Riboflavin   Features of riboflavin deficiency lack specificity. They include angular stomatitis, cheilosis and a heaping up of sebaceous material in the naso-labial folds.

(iv) Niacin   Niacin deficiency (pellagra) is characterized by an erythematous rash on exposed skin which becomes hypertrophied and subsequently atrophies. The gastrointestinal mucosa may be hyperaemic and ulcerated. Diarrhoea and dementia are other features.

(v) Pyridoxine Seborrhoeic dermatitis, glossitis and cheilosis may be accompanied by peripheral neuropathy and, in some children, convulsions. A lymphopenia is associated with anaemia which may occasionally be megaloblastic.

(vi) Vitamin B12 Deficiency of Vitamin B12 has a major impact on the bone marrow and central nervous system. It is commonly responsible for a megaloblastic anaemia recognized on the blood film by macrocytosis, hyperpigmented polymorphonuclear cells, and thrombocytopenia. Rarely it may lead to peripheral neuropathy or the classical syndrome of sub-acute combined degeneration of the cord.

(vii) Vitamin C Vitamin C deficiency causes scurvy. The young baby is irritable with weakness of the legs which are used with reluctance because of pain due to subperiosteal haemorrhage. The adult may complain of aching limbs. Other features include keratosis of the hair follicles and perifollicular haemorrhage, swollen and bleeding gums, and anaemia. Radiological features appear late and are characterized by defects at the corners of the ends of the long bones and a ground glass appearance of the shaft.

(viii) Vitamin D Deficiency of Vitamin D is responsible for rickets and osteomalacia, respectively characterized by reduced calcification of growing and mature bones. The features of rickets are well known. They include enlarged epiphyses, rachitic rosary, kyphoscoliosis and bowing of the limbs with a characteristic waddling gait. Muscular hypotonia contributes to the lordotic posture. The earliest physical sign in a baby is craniotabes due to softening of the occipital bone where the head lies on the pillow. Such features are now extremely rare in developed countries, in contrast to those of osteomalacia which are not rare in the elderly and immigrant population. The adult may complain of bone tenderness, suffer from cramps and exhibit the features of proximal myopathy. Loosers zones, which are bands of demineralization, may be seen on radiograph of long bones.

(ix) Vitamin E Mild deficiency results in haemolytic anaemia, and in more severe deficiency loss of tendon reflexes and pigmentary retinopathy have been described.

(x) Vitamin K Vitamin K deficiency impairs synthesis of coagula-

tion factors leading to haemorrhagic diathesis, evidence of which may be seen from bleeding surgical wounds.

(xi) Folate Folate deficiency causes a megaloblastic anaemia and pancytopenia.

(b) Trace elements

The consequences of deficiency of iodide, iron, calcium and magnesium have long been recognized. Iodide deficiency results in goitre and hypothyroidism in the adult, and cretinism with growth failure and mental retardation in the child. Iron deficiency, which is extremely common, is typically detected by hypochromic microcytic anaemia. Calcium deficiency is often associated with inadequate supplies of Vitamin D and causes impaired skeletal mineralization and severe muscle cramps. Cramps unresponsive to calcium may denote magnesium depletion which is sometimes responsible for cardiac dysrhythmia.

Paradoxically the use of total parenteral nutrition to correct malnutrition and support patients with complete intestinal failure has exposed trace element deficiency syndromes and increased our knowledge of micronutrient requirements. Neutropenia and leukopenia are the reliable markers of copper deficiency and are usually associated with a microcytic hypochromic anaemia. Bone changes may also be evident in children: there is normal growth of cartiliage with the failure of bone deposition in the cartilaginous matrix. Menke's syndrome is a very rare defect of copper absorption which leads to profound copper deficiency in babies. Additional features include sparse brittle hair, arterial and cerebral degeneration.

Patients who receive total parenteral nutrition without zinc supplements develop a psoriasiform rash and diarrhoea. Poor wound healing and susceptibility to fungal and bacterial infections are important features of zinc depletion, and a loss of taste sensation depresses the appetite. Children develop features of dwarfism and hypogonadism, and a congenital defect of zinc absorption causes the syndrome of acrodermatitis enteropathica. This is characterized by a skin rash, hair loss, diarrhoea, paronychia and growth retardation. Features of zinc deficiency occur after a relatively short time because body stores are limited, but a similarly rapid response occurs to replacement therapy.

Selenium deficiency is endemic in a part of China where it is thought to be responsible for a congestive cardiomyopathy called Keshan disease. Prolonged total parential nutrition without selenium supplements has caused myopathy with muscle weakness, pain and elevated creatinine phosphokinase values. Finally trivalent chromium is a component of a glucose tolerance factor and deficiency may lead to glucose intolerance. This also occurs with manganese deficiency which is associated with growth impairment.

4.2.3 NUTRITIONAL DEFICIENCY AND IMMUNITY

Malnutrition has long been associated with susceptibility to infection. However the relevant contribution of malnutrition and overcrowding in the pathogenesis of the frequent epidemics which sweep impoverished communities remains uncertain. Nutritional care has been shown to reduce the incidence of infectious disease in young children. Lymphopenia and thymic atrophy occur in the malnourished but antibody responses are preserved. Complement levels are sometimes reduced and recent attention has been focussed on fibronectin. This facilitates opsonization and declines within a few days of nutrient deficiency. There is defective polymorph function with reduced cell killing. Anergy may relate to protein energy malnutrition or underlying disease such as neoplasia or Crohn's disease.

These developments explain the propensity of the malnourished to post-operative sepsis. Impaired muscle function and immobility are other factors which contribute to the development of respiratory tract infections. Recent interest has focused on the contribution of nutritional impairment to the evolution of opportunistic infections in the acquired immune deficiency syndrome. Nutritional support has been advocated as a means of improving immune defences.

Paradoxically there are some circumstances in which malnutrition appears to confer protection. Falciparum malaria is less severe under famine conditions. This may mean that much of the damage seen in cerebral malaria is attibutable to the host reaction which is suppressed in malnutrition, and the reduced availability of nutrients for the parasites may be relevant. Furthermore, iron deficiency appears to provide some protection against bacterial infection. Fasting has been claimed to improve symptoms of rheumatoid arthritis, but this may reflect the withdrawal of food antigen. Finally over-nutrition has been associated with impaired T cell and neutrophil function, obese children in some studies having a higher incidence of infection.

Deficiency of micronutrients as well as macronutrients is related to the development of impaired immunity. Vitamin A, Vitamin B6 and zinc are important in this respect.

4.3 The causes of malnutrition

Three factors contribute to the development of malnutrition: inadequate diet, impaired absorption and increased nutrient requirements. All three play an important role in the nutritional deficiency seen in hospital practice.

4.3.1 PRIMARY NUTRIENT DEFICIENCY

Primary nutrient deficiency arises when the diet is inadequate and when the appetite is impaired.

(a) Indequate diet

An inadequate diet is the commonest cause of under-nutrition in global terms. Sufficient food is unavailable or inadequately distributed and many people cannot afford to eat satisfactorily. These problems are frequently compounded by lack of knowledge and accentuated by concomitant intestinal disease. In addition to protein energy malnutrition people subsisting on a maize diet of porridge or gruel develop niacin deficiency because food preparation renders niacin unavailable for absorption, and a diet of highly polished rice will lead to thiamin deficiency. Vitamin A deficiency is common in South and East Asia. Thiamin deficiency has also been described in hospital practice following the prolonged administration of intravenous dextrose without vitamin supplementation.

Copper and zinc deficiency occurs in babies as a consequence of prolonged unsupplemented feeding with breast or cow's milk. In the Middle East zinc deficiency is thought to be due to intestinal binding by high fibre phytate rich unleavened bread. The same problem is also responsible for calcium deficiency and may contribute to the development of metabolic bone disease in the United Kingdom immigrant population in whom Vitamin D levels are frequently low. Within the

United Kingdom dietary deficiency is found within other specific groups. Vitamin C and folate deficiency is a common occurrence in the elderly, especially those who live alone or in long-stay institutions. The former may lack the ability, motivation or finance to feed themselves properly. The latter suffer from the problems of institutional cooking which frequently leads to deterioration in food quality and particularly the loss of these vitamins. Similar deficiencies occur in alcoholic subjects in whom the problem of poor diet may be compounded by impaired absorption.

(b) Anorexia

Anorexia is a feature of psychiatric disorders, severe protein energy malnutrition, and specific disease. Depression which may be primary or secondary to underlying disease is an important cause of anorexia and subsequent weight loss. Weight loss is usually the most striking feature of anorexia nervosa in which energy dense foods are assiduously avoided. Severe protein energy malnutrition from whatever cause may lead to appetite impairment which can significantly interfere with management. Such patients are often zinc deficient which leads to impaired taste sensation.

Malignant disease commonly causes anorexia especially if the gastrointestinal tract is involved. Metabolic disorders such as uraemia as well as prolonged sepsis are similarly important reasons for the loss of appetite. Food intake in gastrointestinal disease, for example Crohn's disease, may be reduced not only by anorexia but by the fear of provoking symptoms such as abdominal pain and diarrhoea. Furthermore in gastrointestinal disease the problem of reduced nutrient intake is frequently made worse by malabsorption.

4.3.2 SECONDARY NUTRIENT DEFICIENCY: MALABSORPTION

The physiology of digestion and absorption is discussed in Chapter 2. There are many disorders which are associated with malabsorption, discussion of which is outside the scope of this book. For a comprehensive review the reader is referred to standard textbooks of gastoenterology. The important causes of malabsorption are listed in Table 4.5.

Table 4.5   Important causes of malabsorption

Small bowel disease
   Gluten enteropathy
   Crohn's disease
   Bacterial overgrowth
   Short bowel syndrome
   Radiation enteritis
   Tropical sprue
   Whipples disease
   Intestinal lymphoma
   Scleroderma
   Idiopathic intestinal pseudo-obstruction

Pancreatic disease
   Pancreatic hypoplasia (Schwachman's syndrome)
   Fibrocystic disease
   Chronic pancreatitis

Hepatobiliary disease
   Primary biliary cirrhosis
   Sclerosing cholangitis

Miscellaneous
   Gastric surgery
   Gastrinomas
   Amyloidosis
   Drugs

(a) Intestinal Disease

(i) Gluten enteropathy   Contrary to popular belief the majority of patients with gluten enteropathy do not present with steatorrhoea or even diarrhoea but are identified on the basis of abnormalities in the blood film. Many patients present with isolated folate or iron deficiency reflecting the primary impact on the proximal small intestinal of gluten prior to its degradation. Undoubtedly severe and extensive gluten enteropathy is responsible for protein energy malnutrition, particularly if there is associated ulcerative jejuno-ileitis.

(ii) Crohn's disease   Crohn's disease is an important cause of malnutrition because of several abnormalities, the relative importance of

which varies from patient to patient. Some individuals have extensive small bowel disease which severely impairs intestinal function. In others partial obstruction due to active disease or strictures may encourage bacterial colonization and this also follows the development of intestinal fistulae with which long segments of intestine can be bypassed. More specifically terminal ileal disease impairs the absorption of Vitamin B12 although Vitamin B12 deficiency is uncommon in such subjects. A more significant feature of ileal disease is bile acid malabsorption which contributes to both diarrhoea by the action of bile acid metabolites on the colon and steatorrhoea because of bile acid depletion.

(iii) Bacterial overgrowth in the small intestine The resident intestinal bacterial flora may have a role in the synthesis of vitamins and resistance to specific bacterial pathogens. Overgrowth of this flora however is disadvantageous and may lead to impairment of fat absorption, possibly mediated by bile acid deconjugation and aggravated by mucosal damage. Abnormalities of carbohydrate and protein absorption also occur and often contribute to the malabsorption induced by primary disease. Bacterial colonization of the small intestine is found in children of Third World countries where environmental pollution and impaired immunity due to protein energy malnutrition may be important contributory factors. It commonly arises in patients who are achlorhydric following gastric surgery, due to gastric atrophy, or associated with H_2 antagonist therapy. Blind loops such as jejunal diverticulae, resection of the ileo-caecal valve, and internal fistulae will all predispose to this problem. This syndrome is a recognized reason for malabsorption in the elderly, who are frequently achlorhydric, in the absence of gross intestinal disease. It is important in tropical sprue and radiation enteritis. The latter condition most commonly follows treatment for cervical carcinoma and leads to mucosal damage, fistulae and stricture formation.

(iv) The short bowel syndrome The short bowel syndrome which follows resection for Crohn's disease or ischaemia due to vascular disease or volvulus, leads to malabsorption for many reasons. Gastric hypersecretion, possibly reflecting the loss of gastric inhibitory peptide, imposes a volume load and an unfavourable pH which further impair mixing and enzyme function throughout the residual short intestine. The loss of bile acids reduces micelle formation and,

by definition, there is insufficient intestinal mucosa. Frequently the malabsorption is compounded by dietary insufficiency in an attempt by the patient to prevent unacceptable symptoms of severe diarrhoea.

(b) Pancreatic disease

Pancreatic exocrine insufficiency is a feature of hypoplasia, chronic pancreatitis and cystic fibrosis. The ensuing steatorrhoea can be severe leading to gross malabsorption of fat soluble vitamins and protein. Some patients will also develop deficiencies of Vitamin B12, apparently due to binding with non-intrinsic factor polypeptide: this is reversed by pancreatic enzyme replacement therapy. In advanced disease essential fatty acid deficiency may ensue. The fat malabsorption caused by impaired bile acid delivery and cholestatic liver disease is less severe although the occasional association between primary biliary cirrhosis and gluten enteropathy may lead to more significant nutrient deficiency.

(c) Drugs

Some drugs may impair absorption. Examples include the chelation of iron by Tetracycline and antacid preparations. Cholestyramine used as bile acid binding resin, in the treatment of bile acid diarrhoea or hypercholesterolaemia, will impair the absorption of fat soluble vitamins. Neomycin, an antibiotic used in the treatment of portasystemic encephalopathy, may lead to mucosal damage with associated malabsorption.

4.3.3 INCREASED NUTRIENT REQUIREMENTS

The development of sepsis provokes a series of responses which are discussed more fully in Chapter 2. The liberation of leukocyte endogenous mediator and the enhanced release of catecholamines, glucocorticoids, insulin and glucagon lead to important metabolic changes. There is an overall increase in protein breakdown with a small increase in protein synthesis. Recent studies suggest a reduction of synthesis below the rate of breakdown in muscle and an increase in breakdown with slight reduction in synthesis in visceral tissues. Glucose metabolism is altered with enhanced gluconeogenesis from protein catabolism and increased urinary loss of nitrogen, potassium, phosphate, magnesium and zinc. The consequent negative nitrogen balance is humoraly mediated and cannot be reversed by feeding alone, thus emphasizing the critical importance of treating the underlying infection. Nevertheless there is an increase in the resting metabolic expenditure of up to 50%, rarely up to 100%, in severely burnt and septic patients. This leads to a rapid depletion of the protein and energy stores which require replacement and emphasizes the danger when major sepsis arises as a complication of protein energy malnutrition causing stress in an already depleted patient. Furthermore micronutrient deficiency including zinc and folate may develop if their provision is not increased. The specific amount of these and other micronutrients required under such conditions is unknown.

Drug administration may occasionally be responsible for loss of nutrients. Thiazides and Penicillamine both increase the renal excretion of zinc and Salicylate increases the excretion of Vitamin C. Enzyme inducing drugs, such as Phenytoin, ethanol and Griseofulvin, enhance the metabolism of Vitamin D and folate. Vitamin D deficiency can occur in epileptics for this reasons. Isoniazid, Hydralaxine and D-Penicillamine destroy pyridoxine, and Isoniazid can also induce niacin deficiency after prolonged treatment when the drug replaces niacinamide in NAD. Niacin deficiency can also occur in the carcinoid syndrome because of the diversion of tryptophan to form 5 hydroxtryptamine.

The increased nutrient requirements in patients with chronic renal disease are discussed in Chapter 7. However additional protein may have to be given to patients with proteinuria and those treated by haemodialysis need at least 1 g per kg. Supplemental amino acids or their alpha keto analogues can facilitate protein-restricted diets by extending the range of protein sources.

4.4 Other forms of malnutrition

Surprisingly, examples of dietary insufficiency are not confined to patients in the population of the Third World but may be found in the apparently fit and affluent societies of developed nations. The most notable example which has received widespread publicity is that of dietary fibre. The refinement of carbohydrate food with the exclusion of fibre has been associated with the development of numerous disorders. The increased consumption of sugar and the reduced need for mastication may be important in the development of dental caries.

Reduction in dietary fibre appears to reduce satiety. Satiety may be enhanced by a fibre enriched diet through several mechanisms which include gastric distension and delayed gastric emptying. Thus fibre deficiency could be an important contributory factor in the over-provision of energy. This in turn provokes obesity and enhances the risk of diabetes. Furthermore it is now known that diabetic control can be improved by a fibre enriched diet with which absorption is retarded and insulin stimulation reduced.

Fibre depleted diets have for many years been incriminated in the genesis of ischaemic heart disease and atheroma. Hypotheses linking ischaemic heart disease and dietary fibre include the association between dietary depletion and excess energy consumption, excessive insulin response, and reduced binding and thus clearance of faecal bile acids which are metabolites of cholesterol.

Insufficient fibre is widely regarded as an important cause of numerous gastrointestinal ailments which affect people who consume 'Western' diets and is incriminated in constipation, haemorrhoids, the irritable bowel syndrome, diverticular disease, bowel cancer, and cholelithiasis. The addition of fibre reduces colonic intraluminal pressure and excessive pressure is considered important in the genesis of diverticulae. Fibre is also known to bind bile acid metabolites and these may be important in either promoting bowel cancer or facilitating its development in the presence of other carcinogens. The role of fibre is discussed in Chapter 7.

Malnutrition in developed countries is more frequently a consequence of nutrient excess. Excessive energy consumption in susceptible individuals leads to obesity with its attendant problems of diabetes, hypertension, coronary artery disease, respiratory impairment, osteo-arthrosis and impaired mobility. Recent interest has focused on the potential hazards of high protein diets. Large protein intakes have been incriminated in the development of nephrosclerosis by the induction of hyperfiltration. Conversely protein restriction has been shown to retard the progression of chronic renal impairment.

High sodium consumption has long been debated as a cause of hypertension and current thinking suggests that it may be a dietary factor that elevates blood pressure in susceptible individuals. Finally, excessive phosphate ingestion impairs calcium absorption which may lead to metabolic bone disease. Phosphates are widely distributed but are used increasingly as preservatives and stabilizers in convenience foods and soft drinks.

Until recently most work has focused on the problems caused by under-nutrition. Increasingly the importance of over-nutrition and inappropriate nutrition is being recognized. Much has yet to be learned about these problems and this knowledge is likely to reveal new insights into disease processes and to offer considerable therapeutic potential. This subject is discussed in Chapter 7.

References

Agget, P. J. (1979) Trace elements in medicine. *Hospital Up-Date*, 5, 981–94.

Alleyne, G. A. O., Hay, R. W., Picou, D. I. and Whitehead, R. G. (1977) *Protein Energy Malnutrition*. Arnold, London.

Baker, J. P., Detsky, A. S., Wesson, D. E., Wolman, S. L., Stewart, S., Whitewell, J., Langer, B. and Jeejeebhoy, K. N. (1982) Nutritional assessment. A comparison of clinical judgement and objective measurements. *New England Journal of Medicine*, 306, 969–72.

Bistian, B. R., Blackburn, G. L., Vitale, J., Cochrane, D. and Naylor, J. (1976) Prevalence of malnutrition in general medical patients. *Journal of the American Medical Association*, 235, 1576–80.

Blackburn, G. L. and Thornton, P. A. (1980) Nutritional assessment of the hospitalized patient. *The Medical Clinics of North America*, 63, 1103–15.

Bouchier, I. A. D., Allan, R. N., Hodgson, H. J. F. and Keighley, M. R. B. (eds) (1984) *Textbook of Gastroenterology*. Baillière Tindall, London, Ch. 8, pp. 339–634.

Burch, R. E. and Hahn, H. K. J. (1979) Trace elements in human nutrition. *The Medical Clinics of North America*, 63, 1057–68.

Dickerson, J. W. T. (1981) Vitamins and trace elements in the seriously ill patient. *Acta Chirchurgica Scandinavica*, **Suppl. 507**, 144–50.

Durnin, J. V. G. A. and Wormersley, J. (1974) Body fat assessed from total body density and its estimation from skin fold thickness: measurements on 481 men and women aged from 16 to 72 years. *British Journal of Nutrition*, 32, 77–97.

Haussler, M. R. and McCain, T. A. (1977) Vitamin D metabolism and action. *New England Journal of Medicine*, 297, 974–83 and 1041–50.

Hill, G. L., Blackett, R. L., Pickford, I., Berkinshaw, L., Young, G. A., Warren, J. V., Schorah, C. J. and Morgan, O. B. (1977) Malnutrition in surgical patients. *Lancet*, i, 689–92.

Horowitz, G. D., Groeger, J. S., Legaspi, A. and Lowry, S. F. (1985) The response of fibronectin to different parenteral calorie sources in normal man. *Journal of Parenteral and enteral Nutrition*, 9, 435–42.

McLaren, D. S. (1980) *Nutritional Ophthalmology*, Academic Press, London and New York.

Reinhold, J. G., Lakungarzadek, A., Nasr, K. and Hedayatic, H. (1973) Effects of purified phytate and phytate rich bread upon metabolism of zinc, calcium, phosphorus and nitrogen in Man. *Lancet*, **i**, 283–88.

Rennie, M. J. and Harrison, R. (1984) Effects of injury, disease and malnutrition on protein metabolism in man. *Lancet*, **i**, 323–5.

5

ENTERAL
NUTRITION

Patients may receive nutritional support by the enteral or parenteral routes. The enteral route should be employed whenever the intestinal tract is functional and accessible, and even when enteral nutrition is inadequate because of intestinal failure parenteral nutrition should be supplemental rather than total. Not only is enteral feeding simpler safer and cheaper, but the use of the intestinal tract prevents atrophy and encourages adaption. Enteral feeding is widely available, readily instituted and applicable to the majority of patients who require nutritional support. Enteral nutrition is commonly used to restore or maintain the nutritional status in patients who are unable to eat normally or adequately. Complete nutrient solutions are delivered to the intestinal tract most frequently by the naso-gastric route, occasionally by the oral route, and in selected patients through a feeding jejunostomy. Intubation with a naso-gastric or enteral tube provides more reliable and controlled delivery and overcomes the problem of anorexia which is a feature of protein energy malnutrition as well as underlying disease such as Crohn's disease and neoplasia. The nutrient solutions may be whole protein polymeric diets, chemically defined elemental diets, or special formulations to meet the particular needs of patients with hepatic failure, renal failure or other metabolic disease.

5.1 The role of enteral nutrition

5.1.1 INDICATIONS FOR ENTERAL NUTRITION

Enteral nutrition is helpful in patients who are malnourished, who are unable to eat, in whom nutritional demands are increased following surgery, and in patients who have special requirements.

(a) Patients who are unable to take an oral diet

The administration of liquid feeds through fine bore naso-gastric tubes is invaluable during head and neck surgery and for the management of neurosurgical patients. These tubes can be passed through stenosing oesophageal lesions.

(b) Malnutrition

Malnutrition is common in both medical and surgical practice. Naso-gastric tubes facilitate the reliable delivery of nutrients. They also permit overnight feeding thereby greatly increasing nutrient delivery.

(c) Increased nutrient requirements

Naso-gastric feeding is frequently used to meet the increased requirements of burnt, septic and traumatized patients with nutrient solutions of high energy density.

(d) Post-operative patients

The recognition that small bowel function returns before the resolution of gastric ileus has encouraged the application of feeding jejunostomy for early post-operative nutritional support.

(e) Intestinal failure

Jejunostomy tubes can be used to infuse nutrients distal to enterocutaneous fistulae. Unpalatable chemically defined elemental or peptide diets facilitate the management of distal intestinal fistulae. They are also used in cases of severe malabsorption in association with pancreatic exocrine insufficiency and the short bowel syndrome. Such diets also help to encourage resolution of disease activity in Crohn's disease, a function attributed to hypoallergenicity. Polymeric diets are more commonly used in the treatment of malnutrition associated with intestinal disease.

(f) Miscellaneous applications

The use of special formulation enteral diets is of value in the management of patients with organ failure, a topic which is discussed in Chapter 7. Solutions enriched in branch chain amino acids permit a positive nitrogen balance in patients with chronic liver disease, who are frequently malnourished and prone to portal systemic encephalopathy, without the penalty of deteriorating mental function. Solutions enriched in essential amino acids or keto analogues may facilitate the same objective in patients with renal failure. The use of enteral nutrition in the management of inborn errors of metabolism and food intolerance is described in Chapters 7 and 8 respectively. Minimal residue liquid diets may facilitate pre-operative bowel preparation.

5.1.2 CONTRAINDICATIONS TO ENTERAL FEEDING

A significant number of patients will require parenteral nutrition because features of their illness preclude the use of the enteral route. Contraindications to enteral feeding include:

- Ileus or intestinal obstruction that cannot be bypassed
- Uncontrolled diarrhoea or vomiting
- Multiple or proximal enterocutaneous fistulae when excessive fistulous discharge is provoked by liquid feeds
- The ability to eat an adequate oral diet

5.2 Nutrient solutions

5.2.1 THE RANGE OF COMMERCIAL PRODUCTS

Early liquid diets contained glucose or sucrose as the carbohydrate source combined with amino acids, mineral salts, vitamins and small quantities of fat of high linoleic acid content. They were described as elemental diets. They are relatively expensive to produce, hyperosmolar and unpalatable. They cannot readily be used for oral supplementary feeding. Developments in our understanding of the physiology of digestion and absorption have led to the substitution of peptides and glucose complexes and several such chemically defined diets are currently available. They have a low osmolality and are claimed to give better nitrogen absorption. All provide recommended dietary allowances in two to three litres of solution.

The recognition that intestinal function is not severely impaired in the majority of patients who require enteral nutrition has encouraged the use of polymeric formulas which are liquid feeds prepared from normal foods processed to produce a liquid emulsion or suspension. Carbohydrate sources are partially hydrolysed corn starch or oligo-saccharides and some sucrose, but most contain very little or no lactose. Protein is supplied as calcium and sodium caseinate or soya protein. Fat is derived from soya or corn oil, and in some preparations it is in the form of medium chain triglycerides. Polymeric diets contain no gluten but most provide the recommended micronutrients in two to three litres of solution and 1 kcal per ml of formulation. They have largely replaced chemically defined diets in clinical practice.

Recently some diets have been specially formulated to meet specific needs. Examples include solutions enriched with branch chain amino acids or essential amino acids for patients with portal systemic encephalopathy and renal failure respectively, and high energy and nitrogen density for hypercatabolic patients. In addition to these complete nutrient solutions supplementary feeds are also available and can be used to provide an additional energy source or both energy and protein. They are normally used in conjunction with a conventional oral diet. Paradoxically enteral feeds have also been formulated for the management of obesity. They contain nitrogen electrolytes, minerals and vitamins but very little energy. An example of such a product is Modifast. These preparations will be considered further in Chapter 8.

The recent introduction of many enteral feeding solutions has led to a bewildering array of more than 30 products. Many are similar with minor differences of uncertain clinical significance. The clinician is recommended to become familiar with a limited number of enteral feeds facilitating economies of scale in purchasing costs.

5.2.2 WHOLE PROTEIN FEEDS

The composition of some of the currently available whole protein feeds is summarized in Table 5.1 in which the nutrients contained in two litres of solution are documented. The energy fraction provided by carbohydrate, fat and protein is similar in each product.

(a) Protein

The protein source is usually milk with or without soya protein. There is no milk protein in Fortison.

(b) Fat

Fat is derived from vegetable oil; Clinifeed Iso has some butter fat and Clinifeed 400 egg yolk. In some preparations a portion of the fat is in the form of medium chain triglycerides: 80% of the fat is supplied as medium chain triglycerides in Triosorbon and 20% in Isocal. Medium chain triglycerides are claimed to be more easily absorbed than their long chain equivalents as discussed in Chapter 2. Whereas such preparations may be preferred in patients with severe steatorrhoea, their inclusion results in a bitter taste and occasional symptoms of nausea, abdominal discomfort and diarrhoea.

(c) Carbohydrates

Most of the carbohydrate is in the form of oligosaccarides, mainly maltodextrin, but some products contain disaccharide. Sucrose accounts for a quarter of the carbohydrate in Clinifeed Protein Rich and Ensure.

Lactose is absorbed less efficiently than other disaccharides in patients with intestinal disease and inherited lactase deficiency occurs in 6% of Caucasians and in a high percentage of Asian and African ethnic groups. Unabsorbed lactose which reaches the colon induces osmotic diarrhoea. For these reasons many products such as Isocal, Ensure and Clinifeed LLS are lactose free and relatively small amounts of lactose are present in the rest. One notable exception is Complan, an older milk-based product in which 50% of the carbohydrate is in the form of lactose. In clinical practice the presence of some lactose is of no consequence in the majority of patients.

(d) Electrolytes

Most preparations contain approximately 70 mmol of sodium in two litres. Clinifeed Iso and Fortison Low Sodium respectively provide 30

Table 5.1 Examples of whole protein polymeric feeds: contents of two litres

Feed	Protein g	Fat g	Carbohydrate g	Sodium mmol	Potassium m osml/l	Osmolarity m osml/l	Energy kcal	Protein source	Fat source	Carbohydrate source
Clinifeed (Roussell)										
Clinifeed Iso	56	82	261	30	51	270	2000	Milk/whey	Vegetable oil + butter fat	Corn syrup solids; lactose, sucrose
Clinifeed 400 (Requires dilution)	60	54	220	42	50	306	1600	Milk/whey and egg	Maize oil and soya oil	Corn syrup solids; lactose, sucrose
Clinifeed 500 (Requires dilution)	120	44	280	51	86	567	2000	Milk/whey proteins	Soya oil	Corn syrup solids; lactose, sucrose
Clinifeed LLS (Requires dilution)	90	60	276	28	52	435	2000	Chicken meat, egg yolk, soya protein	Maize oil Soya oil	Maltodextrin No lactose
Ensure (Abbott)										
Ensure	70	70	275	70	76	380	2000	Casein/soya protein isolate	Corn oil	Corn starch Sucrose
Ensure Plus	78	76	284	70	85	500	2130	Casein/soya protein isolate	Corn oil	Corn starch Sucrose
Twocal HN	80	84	206	44	56	533	3800	Casein/soya Protein isolate	Corn oil + Coconut oil	Corn starch Sucrose

Product								Protein source	Fat source	Carbohydrate source
Enrich (Contains fibre)	75	70	306	70	76	402	1900	Casein/soya protein isolate	Corn oil	Corn syrup, sucrose, Soya polysaccharides
Osmolite	70	73	274	45	49	263	2000	Casein/soya protein isolate	MCT (50%), Corn oil + soya oil	Glucose polymers
Enteral (SHS)★ Enteral 400	58	78	288	53	60	330	2000	Whey	Arachis oil MCT oil (25%)	Maltodextrins
Fortison (Cow & Gate) Fortison Standard	80	80	240	70	76	260	2000	Casein	Corn, palm, coconut oils	Maltodextrin Lactose
Fortison Energy Plus	75	98	268	53	57	320	2250	Casein	Corn, palm, coconut oils	Maltodextrin Lactose
Fortison Low Sodium	80	80	240	22	76	220	2000	Casein	Corn, palm, coconut oils	Maltodextrin Lactose
Fortison Soya	80	80	240	70	76	260	2000	Soya	Corn, palm, coconut oils	Maltodextrin Lactose
Fresubin (Fresenius)	76	68	276	66	64	300–340	2000	Casein/soya protein	Sunflower seed oil	Maize, starch, oligopolysaccharides

Table 5.1 continued

Feed	Protein g	Fat g	Carbohydrate g	Sodium mmol	Potassium m osml/l	Osmolarity m osml/l	Energy kcal	Protein source	Fat source	Carbohydrate source
Isocal (Mead & Johnston)	64	84	252	44	64	300	2020	Soya/casein	Soya oil & MCT oil (20% MCT)	Corn syrup solids Oligosaccharides
Liquisorbon (Merck)	80	80	236	90	90	270–340	2000	Whey/casein	Soya oil	Mono–oligopoly-saccharides
Nutrauxil (Kabivitrum)	76	68	276	66	64	350	2000	Casein/soya	Sunflower oil (13% MCT)	Oligopoly-saccharides
Salvimulsin MCT†	96	60	270	80	60	300	2000	Casein Lactalbumin	50% Soya bean 50% MCT	Maltodextrin
Triosorbon (Merck)	81	81	238	85	85	238	2000	Whey/casein	MCT 80% Sunflower oil	Oligo + polysaccharides

*Scientific Hospital Supplies
†Medium chain trnglyccrhides

and 22 mmol of sodium, a property which is of value in patients with sodium retention such as those with ascites and chronic liver disease.

(e) Micronutrients

The micronutrient content varies significantly between different solutions. Unfortunately micronutrient requirements, especially vitamin requirements, are unknown in many disease states but are thought to be greater than in healthy subjects. The folate content is low in Triosorbon, and Vitamin C content is high in Ensure and Isocal. This latter also provides a large amount of Vitamin A. The content of manganese, copper and zinc appears inadequate in Triosorbon and Nutrauxil, and is lower in the Clinifeed preparations than in Isocal or Ensure.

(f) Osmolality

Hyperosmolar solutions are prone to draw water into the proximal small bowel and thus induce diarrhoea. Whereas the relevance of osmolality to the development of diarrhoea, at least in the range associated with commercial enteral feeds, has been disputed, it is customary to dilute solutions with osmolarities in excess of 300 m osm/l at the onset of feeding. Continuous feeding rather than bolus feeding is also important.

(g) Taste

When these solutions are being used for supplementary oral feeding taste is important. Flavours may have to be added to disguise the bitterness of medium chain triglycerides, and the distortion of the sense of taste in ill patients particularly those with neoplastic disease must be considered. The vanilla flavour of Ensure and Clinifeed, which is attractive to healthy subjects, may be unacceptable to such patients.

(h) 'Home brew'

Finally many dietetic departments produce their own whole protein liquid feeds. The apparent advantage of the lower cost of the ingredients may be outweighed by their labour intensive production and limited shelf life. Such solutions are usually more viscous and block fine bore feeding tubes, and they may also be a significant source of infection.

5.2.3 PEPTIDE BASED FEEDS

Whole protein polymeric diets require digestion before absorption so they are less suitable for patients with severe digestive abnormalities such as the short bowel syndrome, pancreatic exocrine insufficiency, and cystic fibrosis. Elemental diets are preferred for such patients. Early elemental diets contained amino acid solutions similar to those used in parenteral nutrition. Recent research into the mechanism of digestion and absorption has suggested that di and tri-peptides are absorbed more rapidly than amino acid solutions, although the design of these studies and the validity of their conclusions have been criticized. Nevertheless several peptide based formulas are now available and are promoted for the management of patients with severe digestive impairment described above. These products are generally more palatable and have a lower osmolarity than the amino acid solutions. They are summarized in Table 5.2.

5.2.4 AMINO ACID BASED (ELEMENTAL) FEEDS

Preparations such as Vivonex were originally marketed for the management of patients with severe digestive and absorptive disorders and are summarized in Table 5.3. Vivonex itself has a very low fat content which is supplied as purified sunflower oil. This may be a significant advantage in patients with severe malabsorption. Flexical and Elemental 028 share with Vivonex a relatively low nitrogen content: a high nitrogen form of Vivonex is available but the osmolarity is also high.

Other indications for the use of elemental diets include bile acid induced diarrhoea and the investigation and management of food allergy. The apparent efficacy of elemental diets in the management of Crohn's disease may in part relate to hypo-allergenicity permitting resolution of disease activity. Whereas preliminary studies are encouraging, further evaluation of the role of these agents in this context is required.

Unless specifically indicated, elemental diets should not be used. They are less palatable and more expensive than peptide diets which in

Table 5.2 Examples of peptide based feeds: contents of two litres

Feed	Protein g	Fat g	Carbohydrate g	Sodium mmol	Potassium m osml/l	Osmolarity m osml/l	Energy kcal	Protein source	Fat source	Carbohydrate source
Nutranel (Roussell)	80	20	372	40	72	410	2000	Hydrolysate of whey 80–85% peptide 15–20% amino acids	Corn oil MCT oil (50%)	Maltodextrin
Peptisorbon (Merck)	81	26	350	120	60	400	2000	Hydrolysate of lactalbumin 80% oligopeptide 20% amino acid	MCT (60%) Sunflower oil	Maltodextrin
Peptide 2+ (SHS)	56	72	252	37	52	288	1800	Hydrolysate of meat + soya protein as peptides	Coconut, animal fat, groundnut oil 35% MCT	Maltodextrin
MCT Peptide 2+ (SHS)	56	75	250	54	52	360	1840	Hydrolysed meat + soya protein as peptides	Coconut oil, linoleic acid 83% MCT	Maltodextrin
Reabilan (Roussell)	63	78	263	54	56	300	2000	Hydrolysate of whey + casein as small peptides	Evening primrose Soya oil	Maltodextrin Starch
Salvipeptid (MCP Pharmaceuticals)	67	24	380	120	60	450	2000	Hydrolysed lactalbumin 65% oligo-peptide 25% amino acid 10% polypeptides	Soya bean oil	Maltodextrin

Table 5.3 Examples of amino acid based feeds: contents of two litres

Feed	Protein g	Fat g	Carbohydrate g	Sodium mmol	Potassium m osml/l	Osmolarity m osml/l	Energy k cal	Protein source	Fat source	Carbohydrate source
Elemental 028 (SHS)	40	27	312	52	47	450	1600	Amino acids	Arachis oil	Maltodextrin
Flexical (Mead-Johnston)	45	68	304	30	64	550	2000	Hydrolysed casein as peptides and amino acids	Soya oil MCT	Glucose oligosaccharides and tapioca starch
Vivonex Standard (Eaton Lab)	41	3	460	75	60	610	2000	Amino acids	Purified sunflower oil	Glucose oligosaccharides
Vivonex H.N. (Eaton Lab)	88	2	422	70	37	800	2000	Amino acids	Purified sunflower oil	Glucose oligosaccharides

turn are twice as expensive as polymeric diets. However it is worth noting that one exception is Vivonex which is much cheaper than Elemental 028 and not much more expensive than some polymeric formulations.

5.2.5 SPECIAL FORMULATIONS

(a) Hypercatabolic patients

Patients who are stressed, septic, traumatized or burnt have greater nutritional requirements. Previously it was customary to provide very large amounts of energy and nitrogen but the application of modern investigative techniques has demonstrated requirements lower than previously postulated. Nevertheless they are frequently increased by up to 50% and occasionally up to 100% in severely burnt patients. Traditionally such needs were supplied using larger volumes of protein feed or a high nitrogen protein feed with the addition of energy supplements such as Caloreen which are described in Section 5.2.6. Newer diets with energy density increased from 1 kcal/ml to 1.5–2 kcal/ml and higher nitrogen content are now available, for example Twocal HN.

Some authorities claim that branch chain enriched solutions improve nitrogen balance in hypercatabolic patients. This has not been borne out by all studies and further work is required before such solutions can be recommended for routine use in this context. However branch chain enriched feeds have recently been introduced for the management of hypercatabolic patients. One example is Stress Nutril. This product also contains additional carnitine which is required for the entry of long chain triglycerides into mitochondria.

(b) Chronic liver disease and portal systemic encephalopathy

There is more support for the role of branch chain enriched amino acid solutions in the management of patients with portal systemic encephalopathy and chronic liver disease, in whom their use permits nutritional support without increasing neurological impairment. Hepataid is an early example of such a preparation but it contains a large amount of glucose which can cause problems with glucose intolerance, a feature in many of these patients. Other such preparations include Hepato-Nutril and Hepatomine.

(c) Renal failure

Formulations enriched in essential amino acids are available for use in patients with chronic renal failure (Nephro-Nutril and Dialamine). These are often used as dietary supplements to expand the range of available protein sources.

(d) Respiratory failure

Recent interest has focused on the limited tolerance of glucose in stressed patients, a subject which is discussed more fully in Chapter 6. Attempts to meet the entire energy requirement with glucose in such patients may increase carbon dioxide production and oxygen consumption. This can be unacceptable in patients with respiratory impairment. A diet has been formulated with a reduced ratio of carbohydrate to fat for use in these circumstances (Pulmocare).

(e) Inborn errors of metabolism

Preparations with special amino acid formulation for use in patients with inborn errors of metabolism will be mentioned in Chapter 7.

5.2.6 SUPPLEMENTARY FEEDS

Supplementary feeds can be used to provide an additional energy source or both energy and protein. They are nutritionally incomplete and normally complement an oral diet. Preparations providing energy include Hycal, Caloreen, Maxijul and Duocal are in a liquid or powder form. Protein and energy supplements include Complan, Build-Up and Fortimel or locally prepared high protein 'drinks' supplied from the diet kitchen.

5.3 Methods of enteral feeding

Nutrient solutions may be administered by the oral route, by the naso-gastric route, or by a variety of other methods including the naso-enteral tube, pharyngostomy, gastrostomy or jejunostomy. These methods are not mutually exclusive and in the absence of contraindications patients should be encouraged or allowed to eat normal food to complement their enteral feeding.

5.3.1 ORAL FEEDING

Where possible the patient is encouraged to eat a ward diet or provided with a special diet according to needs or preferences. The nutritional content may be increased by addition of the energy or protein supplements previously described. Alternatively when very little conventional diet is taken supplementation with whole protein polymeric liquid feeds is preferred to provide a more complete nutrient spectrum. The choice will depend upon local availability and taste preferences.

The technique of sip feeding is particularly useful for the anorectic individual. A glass of liquid feed is placed by the bed and the patient is invited to regard it as a 'gin and tonic': constant sipping throughout the day is interrupted for an hour before each meal. The provision of a straw may be more appealing for children and enable adults to drink the liquid with minimal appreciation of taste.

Oral feeding in this way is simple, cheap and safe but it requires a co-operative patient and the encouragement of a diligent nurse. There is uncertainty about the amount of nutrient consumed and intake is often inadequate particularly as the time when the patient sleeps is unavailable for nutritional support. For these reasons the naso-gastric route is often employed even when patients are able to eat normally.

5.3.2 NASO-GASTRIC FEEDING

Naso-gastric feeding is the commonest method of delivering nutritional support. Containers of nutrient solutions are attached to naso-gastric tubes through which the feed is pumped or infused as shown in Figure 5.1. Numerous delivery systems are currently available.

(a) Equipment for naso-gastric feeding

(i) Naso-gastric tubes The traditional Ryles tube used for 'drip and suck' and previously for bolus feeding is unacceptable as it may damage the oesophagus. Modern naso-gastric tubes are much narrower, the smallest such as the Clinifeed tube have internal diameters of 1 mm and slightly larger tubes, such as the Corpak-Silk, permit gastric aspiration without causing discomfort. Most are radio-opaque. Some have flexible guidewires to facilitate placement, others

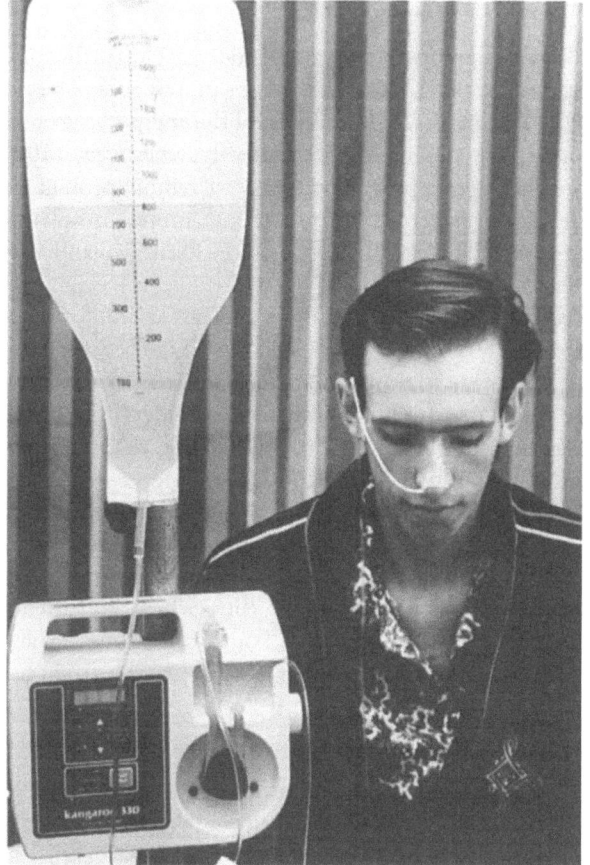

Figure 5.1 Patient receiving naso-gastric feeding

have mercury weighted tips. The latter are more expensive but advantageous in patients with endo-tracheal tubes, oesophageal strictures, or for naso-enteral feeding. Most of the tubes are made of polyvinyl chloride. This may stiffen with time and some manufacturers recommend the tubes are changed every 10 days. The more expensive polyurethane or silicon tubes are preferred when prolonged use is anticipated, for example in neurosurgical patients. The characteristics of some of the naso-gastric tubes are shown in Table 5.4. The Clinifeed tube is very widely used. Multilumen tubes are also avail-

Table 5.4 Some examples of enteral feeding tubes

Tube	Connection	Material	End
Clinifeed	Reversed luer	Polyvinyl chloride	Plain
Dobhoff	Luer	Polyurethane	Side holes, weighted
Portex	Reversed luer	Polyvinyl chloride	Side holes
Corpak-Silk	Reversed luer	Polyurethane	Side holes, bullet tip
Vygon	Reversed luer	Silicone	Side holes
Vygon	Reversed luer	Polyvinyl chloride	Plain

able. They are potentially useful in the post-operative patient and allow simultaneous gastric aspiration and duodenal feeding.

(ii) Reservoirs and administration sets Many manufacturers supply reservoirs and administration sets. The most satisfactory equipment consists of a collapsible bag with integral or separate giving sets preferably with luer connections. Equipment can be selected according to local requirements. Whereas an infusion pump is not so important for enteral feeding as for parenteral nutrition, excessive flow rates may induce diarrhoea and vomiting with the risk of inhalation. Conversely slow flow rates may cause the tube to block. For

Table 5.5 Examples of pumps for enteral feeding

Pump	Manufacturer
Clinifeed	Roussel
Flexiflow	Abbott
Fortison	Cow and Gate
Kangaroo	Cheeseborough Ponds

these reasons many clinicians prefer to control the infusion by using a pump and this is especially important for the patient receiving home nocturnal naso-enteral hyperalimentation. A variety of pumps are now commercially available, and some are listed in Table 5.5. They deliver a reasonable flow range with acceptable accuracy. The use of some conventional peristaltic pumps is inadvisable because they are capable of generating high pressures in the event of occlusion.

(b) Insertion of the naso-gastric catheter

This is readily achieved in co-operative patients who are able to swallow. The patient should be in a sitting position but should not lean forward. The required length of tube is estimated and lubricated with water and a guidewire is inserted. The tube is then passed through the nostril into the naso-pharynx and advanced into the stomach while the patient swallows sips of water. Coughing may indicate tracheal intubation and under these circumstances the tube is withdrawn and reinserted.

An endoscopic method may be employed for the intubation of patients who are unable to swallow. Topical anaesthesia is applied to the oropharynx and the distal end of the tube is passed through the nostril. When it is visible in the oropharynx the stiffening wire is removed, the tube is grasped with forceps and pulled out through the mouth when the distal 5 cm are placed in the biopsy channel of an endoscope. The endoscope is inserted into the stomach where the tube is dislodged using biopsy forceps.

Confirmation of the tube position is important and can be achieved by auscultation of the epigastrium while air is instilled or in the case of larger tubes by gastric aspiration. Radiological confirmation of position is preferred in drowsy or comatose patients.

(c) Methods of feeding

Feeds should be given by the continous drip technique using a feed reservoir and a giving set attached to a fine bore catheter. The use of an infusion pump is desirable but in most circumstances it is not essential. This method has superseded the bolus feeding technique which is more likely to produce diarrhoea and is more demanding on nursing time. Furthermore continuous infusion permits nocturnal feeding thus allowing increased nutrient provision.

Naso-gastric feeds are introduced slowly in a dilute form to avoid symptoms of intolerance such as diarrhoea and abdominal distention. Slow introduction is particularly important in the patient who has not been fed enterally for a few weeks when intestinal atrophy will reduce tolerance. Tolerance of water is established first, subsequently quarter, half and then full strength feeds are introduced on successive days. This process is retarded in the presence of intolerance. The need for such starter regimes has been disputed by some authorities when using solutions with the osmolarity of commercially available preparations, diarrhoea being attributed to the coincidental use of antibiotic therapy rather then the osmolarity of the solution.

As with earlier studies on parenteral feeding the metabolic advantages of cyclical infusion enteral therapy have recently been advocated. The practical importance of intermittent infusion remains to be demonstrated. Disadvantages of the intermittent technique include a loss of infusion time and thus nutrient delivery or the need for increased infusion rate which may not be tolerated.

This method of nutrient delivery overcomes the problem of

anorexia and removes a responsibility of nutrient ingestion from the reluctant patient and busy nursing staff. It allows utilization of the intestinal tract when the patient is resting or sleeping, is simple and generally well tolerated. Potential disadvantages include the risk of inhalation of nutrient with gastro-oesophageal reflux and tube displacement by restless or confused patients.

(d) Home nocturnal naso-gastric hyperalimentation

Co-operative patients with satisfactory domestic circumstances and supportive relatives may receive naso-gastric nutrition at home. Home nocturnal naso-gastric feeding is a particularly useful technique in which the patient is taught to pass a fine bore naso-gastric tube each night. The nutrient solution is infused during sleep and the tube is removed the following morning. Such patients live normal lives during the day taking an oral diet if possible.

Indications for this technique include chronic malnutrition associated with neoplastic disease, cystic fibrosis or intestinal disease. Crohn's disease is a particularly common reason for such treatment which enables the correction of malnutrition, management of growth failure, and delivery of unpalatable nutrients such as Vivonex (used by some authorities for its hypoallergenic properties).

Patients are supplied with a new naso-gastric tube each night. New delivery tubes should be used on each occasion but reservoirs may be reused for a few days provided they are cleaned after use. The Clinifeed System 3 has proved very satisfactory for this purpose. A pump is strongly recommended in the home situation even though fine bore catheters offer some protection against rapid infusion with the attendant risks of gastric distension and inhalation. The small battery-operated frusenius pump provides a portable system.

Home nocturnal naso-gastric feeding should be considered in all patients with chronic intestinal failure. It may avoid the need for home parenteral nutrition which is infinitely more expensive and more hazardous.

5.3.3 OTHER ENTERAL FEEDING METHODS

(a) Naso-jejunal feeding

This method may be preferred in patients with functional or partial anatomical gastric outlet obstruction, those with duodenal or gastric fistulae, and to minimize oesophageal reflux and aspiration in patients who are comatose or who have neurological deficits such as motor neurone disease. It may also be advantageous in post-operative patients with normal small bowel motility but persisting gastric ileus. Weighted catheters are preferred but often fail to pass into the appropriate position. Endoscopic methods may be useful for catheter placement as previously described. Multi-lumen balloon naso-enteric tubes permit oesophageal aspiration as well as simultaneous aspiration of the stomach and feeding into the duodenum. The facility for gastric decompression is particularly valuable in the post-operative situation.

(b) Pharyngostomy and oesophagostomy

These techniques are applied when naso-pharyngeal intubation is not tolerated or contraindicated and are particularly useful for head and neck operations and following oesophagogastrectomy. Pharyngostomy and cervical oesophagostomy are simple procedures which can be performed under local anaesthesia. A feeding tube is placed through the stoma. Skin irritation around the stoma is a minor problem, whereas pulmonary aspiration and oesophageal damage are more serious. There have been reports of arterial erosion and fatal haemorrhage in patients with irradiated necks. A new oesophagostomy tube with a silicon flange collar and wide lumen appears to be advantageous in clinical use.

(c) Gastrostomy

This provides ready access to the stomach, bypassing oesophageal disease. The procedure is more difficult and great care is required to avoid peritonitis due to gastric leakage, so the insertion site through the gastrointestinal wall must be carefully sutured. Most techniques involve the use of a tube. Problems include tube displacement, skin irritation, or peritonitis due to the leak of gastric contents. Conventional gastrostomies are no longer widely employed but the recently described technique of percutaneous endoscopic gastrostomy may prove useful. With the patient lying on their back an assistant probes the anterior abdominal wall and the point of maximum gastric indentation, viewed through an endoscope, is marked. After the instillation of local anaesthetic an intravenous needle and cannula is pushed through a 1 cm skin incision and through the wall of the stomach which is supported by an open polypectomy snare. The needle is removed, thread is inserted through the cannula, grasped by the snare and pulled out through the mouth by withdrawing the endoscope. This end of the thread is then tied through a slit in a feeding cannula which is then pulled back through the anterior abdominal wall. A flange retains the other end of the cannula in the stomach. Clearly this is a relatively simple technique which can be achieved without general anaesthetic but is only suitable for thin patients. The value of endoscopic percutaneous gastrostomy awaits further experience.

(d) Jejunostomy

Needle catheter jejunostomy involves the percutaneous introduction of a fine catheter through a 14 gauge needle into the bowel along an intramural tunnel. It is secured to the bowel with a suture, and new catheters have dacron cuffs to facilitate anchorage in the subcutaneous tunnel. This technique may be useful for the management of patients with proximal obstruction or fistulae or when the stomach is absent.

Advantages over gastrostomy include less stomal leakage and skin irritation, less gastric and pancreatic secretion, reduced nausea, vomiting and bloating, and a reduced risk of aspiration. Fine tube jejunostomy has been used to feed ambulant patients including those with cystic fibrosis in a domiciliary setting. However it is inappropriate for patients with peritonitis, ascites, Crohn's disease and obesity. Complications include tube displacement, peritonitis and small bowel fistulization.

5.4 Complications of enteral feeding

The complications of enteral feeding may be considered in three groups, those related to the route of delivery, gastrointestinal side-effects, and metabolic complications. Enteral feeding is generally safer than parenteral nutrition.

5.4.1 COMPLICATIONS OF NUTRIENT DELIVERY

(a) Oesophageal damage

The previously reported complications of naso-gastric intubation with large bore Ryle's tubes including sinusitis, oesophagitis and oesophageal stricture, have not been reported with fine bore tubes. However fine bore naso-gastric tubes readily pass into the trachea and are more readily removed by the patient.

(b) Inhalation

Naso-gastric feeding may lead to oesophageal reflux and in some patients this can cause inhalational pneumonia.

(c) Stomal leakage

Gastrostomy and jejunostomy may be associated with nutrient leakage causing peritonitis or skin irritation.

(d) Catheter occlusion

Fine bore feeding tubes occasionally become occluded, usually when viscous home made nutrient preparations are infused.

(e) Inappropriate delivery

There have been reports of the intravenous administration of enteral feeds which may be fatal. The use of feeding tubes and giving sets with reversed luer locks ensures that the enteral and parenteral systems are incompatible.

5.4.2 GASTROINTESTINAL SIDE-EFFECTS

Nausea, abdominal distension, pain and diarrhoea are the most frequent side-effects which have been reported in up to 25% of patients. These features are usually attributed to the delivery of hypertonic solutions into the small intestine. Tolerance may be improved by the use of diluted starter regimes, the avoidance of bolus feeding and the careful control of the rate of infusion using an appropriate pump. Cautious infusion is particularly important in patients who are being weaned from total parenteral nutrition especially if there has been a prolonged period of bowel rest during which mucosal atrophy will have occurred.

Other factors incriminated in the development of diarrhoea include the use of lactose containing feeds and feeds with bacterial contamination. Both may be avoided with sterilized commercial feeds. Diarrhoea is sometimes associated with concomitant antimicrobial therapy.

5.4.3 METABOLIC COMPLICATIONS

The development of metabolic complications may reflect pre-existing deficiencies, the stress of active disease or trauma or the gradual introduction of enteral feeds using dilute solutions when the need for additional electrolyte provision may be overlooked. The more common metabolic complications include hyperglycaemia, hypokalaemia and hypophosphataemia. Such problems are prevented or corrected by careful monitoring. Minor abnormalities of liver function tests, particularly with alkaline phosphatase and gamma glutamyl transpeptidase, are observed in up to 40% of patients. This is often due to hepatic steatosis and enzyme values return to normal when treatment is stopped. Significant disturbance of liver function is more commonly related to the underlying disease rather than this form of nutritional therapy.

5.5 Patient monitoring

Careful patient monitoring is essential for the recognition of malnutrition, characterization of nutrient requirements, assessment of response to treatment, and the prevention of complications.

The use of clinical, anthropometric and biochemical indices in the diagnosis of malnutrition is discussed in Chapter 3, and a detailed regime for monitoring patients who are receiving parenteral nutrition is described in Chapter 6. In most patients monitoring does not need to be as stringent during enteral nutrition.

Patients should be fully assessed prior to the initiation of therapy and daily measurements of fluid balance, weight, blood glucose, urea and electrolytes are required in the early phase of treatment. Weekly measurement of haemoglobin, calcium, phosphate, zinc, magnesium, albumin and liver function tests may suffice unless the patient is metabolically unstable with fluctuating requirements. The frequency of urine collections for nitrogen balance studies will be determined by the clinical needs of the patient.

5.6 The cost of enteral nutrition

Enteral feeding is very much cheaper than parenteral nutrition because the cost of equipment and nutrient solutions is much lower and it makes no significant demands on pharmacy or nursing time. Costs will be determined by the amount and nature of nutrients required and the type of nutritional support. Naso-gastric tubes remain in position for several weeks in hospital patients whereas those receiving home nocturnal naso-gastric hyperalimentation are provided with a new tube each night. The reservoirs and delivery sets can be reused and renewed twice weekly in both groups.

Whole protein feeds are significantly cheaper. The nutrient cost of providing an average 2000 kcal feed (8.4 MJ) is approximately £4.00 to £5.00 per day. Special preparations containing fibre or medium chain triglycerides are more expensive. Peptide based feeds cost two to three times as much and the same applies to some elemental feeds although the original preparation Vivonex is relatively cheap. The cost of the reservoir giving set and naso-gastric tubes may add a further £2.00 to £3.00 per day. The pumps cost £200 to £300. Consequently it is possible to provide adequate enteral nutrition for less than £7.00 per day. In contrast parenteral nutrition costs over £70.00 per day.

References

Brown, J. (1981) Enteral feeds and delivery systems. *British Journal of Hospital Medicine*, **26**, 168–75.

Dunn, E. L., Moore, E. E. and Bohus, R. W. (1980) Immediate post-operative feeding following massive abdominal trauma: the catheter jejunostomy. *Journal of Parenteral and Enteral Nutrition*, **4**, 393–5.

Elia, M. (1982) The effects of nitrogen and energy intake on the metabolism of normal, depleted and injured man. Considerations for practical nutritional support. *Clinical Nutrition*, **1**, 173–92.

Hughes, E. C. (1978) Use of a chemically defined diet in the diagnosis of food sensitivities and the determination of offending foods. *Annals of Allergy*, **40**, 393–8.

Keighley, M. R. B., Mogg, B., Bentley, S. and Allan, C. (1982) 'Home brew' compared with commercial preparations for enteral feeding. *British Medical Journal*, **284**, 163.

Keohane, P. P., Attrill, H. and Silk, D. B. A. (1983) Endoscopic placement of fine bore naso-gastric and naso-enteral feeding tubes. *Clinical Nutrition.* **1**, 245–7.

Keohane, P. P., Attrill, H., Love, M., Frost, P. and Silk, D. B. A. (1984) Relation between osmolality of diet and gastrointestinal side-effects in enteral nutrition. *British Medical Journal*, **288**, 678–80.

Meguid, M. M., Eldar, S. and Wahba, A. (1985) The delivery of nutritional support. A pot-pourri of new devices and methods. *Cancer*, **55**, 278–89.

Ó'Moráin, C., Segal, A. W. and Levi, A. J. (1984) Elemental diet as primary treatment of acute Crohn's disease: a controlled trial. *British Medical Journal*, **288**, 1859–63.

Russell, R. I. (1985) Elemental diets: part 1. Their properties and metabolic effects. *Current Concepts in Gastroenterology*, **3**, 10–16.

Ryan, J. A. and Page, C. P. (1984) Intrajejunal feeding: development and current status. *Journal of Parenteral and Enteral Nutrition*, **8**, 187–98.

Silk, D. B. A., Fairclough, P. D. and Clark, M. L. (1980) The use of a peptide rather than a free amino acid nitrogen source in chronically defined elemental diets. *Journal of Parenteral and Enteral Nutrition*, **4**, 548–52.

Silk, D. B. A. (1983) *Enteral Feeding in Nutritional Support in Hospital Practice*, Blackwell Scientific Publications, Oxford, pp. 68–101.

6

PARENTERAL NUTRITION

Abdominal disease, surgery and trauma are common problems which may lead to the inadequacy or unavailability of the intestinal tract. Parenteral nutrition is essential under these circumstances to prevent or alleviate malnutrition which increases morbidity and mortality by impaired immunity and wound healing.

Parenteral nutrition with dextrose as an energy substrate was described in 1911. Lipid became available for intravenous administration after the development of an emulsion from soya bean oil and egg phosphlipid. Following the early use of protein hydrolysates which were incompletely metabolized, solutions of crystalline laevo amino acids were synthesized and found to be efficiently utilized. During the last 20 years further important developments have occurred. These include knowledge of micronutrient requirements and nutrient needs during stress, and improved methods of nutrient delivery. Consequently parenteral nutrition today is simple, relatively safe and widely applicable. It has greatly facilitated the management of patients with intestinal failure.

6.1 Indications for parenteral nutrition

Parenteral nutrition is potentially hazardous and very expensive, and it imposes significant demands on pharmacy and nursing resources. For these reasons it should be employed only when adequate nutrition cannot be achieved or maintained by the enteral route. Parenteral nutrition is indicated in patients with gastrointestinal failure, when bowel rest is required, and occasionally in hypercatabolic states.

6.1.1 INTESTINAL FAILURE

(a) Short bowel syndrome

Intestinal failure is a feature of the short bowel syndrome following intestinal resection for Crohn's disease, volvulus, or mesenteric vascular disease.

(b) Extensive intestinal disease

This occurs in patients who have extensive Crohn's disease or radiation enteritis, or enterocutaneous fistulae which may complicate a variety of diseases.

(c) Motility disorders

Uncommon causes include motility disorders such as idiopathic intestinal pseudo-obstruction and scleroderma. In patients with scleroderma intestinal failure is usually associated with severe disease of other organ systems.

6.1.2 BOWEL REST

(a) Intestinal surgery

Bowel rest is essential after some forms of surgery, and parenteral nutrition should be give to patients in whom enteral nutrition is unlikely to be available for more than five days or early in the presence of major surgery, sepsis, or preceding malnutrition.

(b) Pancreatitis

Bowel rest has also been advocated for acute pancreatitis thus avoiding pancreatic stimulation by enteral feeding. Not only may it speed the resolution of an acute pancreatitis, it is clearly necessary when severe pancreatitis is associated with an ileus and it may also be needed to correct pre-existing malnutrition especially in alcoholic patients.

(c) Crohn's disease

Recently bowel rest therapy has been used in the management of acute Crohn's disease. It has been suggested that allergens contained in the diet either provoke or at least aggravate mucosal inflammation. Whereas parenteral nutrition will facilitate the resolution of disease activity and correct malnutrition, in some patients the same objectives may be achieved by the use of elemental diets such as Vivonex.

6.1.3 HYPERCATABOLIC STATES

Until recently the hypercatabolic patient with burns, sepsis or trauma was considered to have very large nutrient requirements exceeding the capacity of the intestinal tract. It was not unusual for such patients to receive 6000 kcal (25 MJ) per day. However energy expenditure when measured by modern techniques has been found to be much lower. With the exception of extensive burns very few patients expend more than 45 kcal/kg (0.19 MJ/kg). Nevertheless, parenteral nutrition may still be expedient because of gastroparesis, ileus and large fluid requirements.

6.1.4 MISCELLANEOUS DISORDERS

(a) Malignant disease

Parenteral nutrition is widely applied in the management of patients with neoplastic disease many of whom suffer from severe malnutrition. Such treatment may be appropriate in patients with gastrointestinal tumours to facilitate definitive treatment but the general application of this therapy is difficult to justify unless the enteral route is impaired or unavailable for some other reason, possibly as a result of cytotoxic chemotherapy. Claims that parenteral nutrition enhances response to chemotherapy while offering protection against adverse reactions require further substantiation.

(b) Growth retardation

Parenteral nutrition has been shown to induce growth in developmentally retarded patients with Crohn's disease. Such treatment can be very successful but it should only be applied to patients in whom the inadequancy of the enteral route is established.

Wherever possible parenteral nutrition should be used as an adjunct rather than an alternative to enteral feeding. Supplemental rather than total parenteral nutrition prevents atrophy of the small intestinal mucosa and enteral feeding encourages adaption in the short bowel syndrome.

6.2 Parenteral nutrients

The nutrients required are shown in Table 6.1. When patients need total rather than supplemental parenteral nutrition great care must be taken to ensure the adequacy of nutrient provision. This relates not only to the energy and nitrogen needs but also to essential fatty acids, electrolytes and trace elements. Account must be taken of recommended daily requirements and of any additional losses the patient may sustain, for example through enterocutaneous fistulae. Nutrients should be infused simultaneously to facilitate optimum utilization. Special requirements which occur in organ failure or metabolic disease will be considered in Chapter 7.

6.2.1 ENERGY

(a) Dextrose

Available energy sources are given in Table 6.2. Dextrose is cheap and readily metabolized, but concentrated solutions are hypertonic and must be delivered via the central vein.

The minimum daily requirement of dextrose is approximately 100 g, and administration of excess dextrose results in lipogenesis with a marked increase in carbon dioxide production and a lesser increase in oxygen consumption. In the short-term the development of hepatic steatosis may be of no consequence but the increased respiratory demand can create problems for patients who are being weaned off artificial ventilation. Furthermore studies indicate that stressed patients such as those with extensive burns or undergoing

Table 6.1 Nutrient requirements

Dextrose
Lipid
Amino acids
Electrolytes
Trace elements
Vitamins
Water

Table 6.2 Energy sources

Recommended	Not recommended
Dextrose	Fructose
Intralipid	Sorbitol
	Xylitol
	Ethanol

major surgery have a reduced capacity for glucose beyond which increases in protein synthesis and direct oxidation no longer occur. This limit may be as low as 5 mg/kg per minute in burn patients and 6–7 mg per kg per minute in general surgical patients.

The normal resting metabolic expenditure is 30 kcal/kg per 24 hours (0.13 MJ per 24 hours) in males. This may be reduced by 25% in chronic starvation or when respiratory energy expenditure is removed by ventilatory support. Conversely it may increase by 10% after elective abdominal surgery and by 25% following major surgery. Much larger increases follow burns i.e. 25% to 50% with 30% burns and 100% for 70% burns. Consequently it may not be desirable to meet all energy requirements with dextrose for reasons which have previously been outlined. The balance of energy needs may be infused as lipid.

(b) Lipid

A soya oil emulsion stabilized with egg yolk phosphatide (Intralipid) has been available for more than 20 years. Similar products have been introduced more recently e.g. Travomulsion. The advantages of lipid as an energy source include high energy density (9 kcal/g, 0.038 MJ/g), isotonicity even with 20% Intralipid which facilitates peripheral venous administration, and the provision of essential fatty acids.

Daily inspection of the serum to establish lipid clearance is essential when initiating therapy. In spite of reports of the *in vitro* agglutination of Intralipid by the sera of acutely ill patients, probably precipitated by C-reactive protein, and autopsy findings of micro-embolism which could be caused by Intralipid agglutination, this product is relatively safe given appropriate monitoring. Occasionally patients develop a febrile reaction and this is usually associated with the 20% solution. Reports of impairment of monocyte and neutrophil function in patients who receive Intralipid are of uncertain clinical significance and it must be remembered that hyperglycaemia, which is more likely to develop when glucose is used as a sole energy source, also impairs immune function.

Intralipid is used increasingly as an energy source in conjunction with glucose following the recognition of limited glucose tolerance in some patients and the realization that Intralipid can be safely compounded with other nutrients in ethylene vinyl acetate bags. In most patients this dual energy source promotes nitrogen retention as effectively as dextrose alone with less fluid retention.

When Intralipid is not employed as an energy source it should be given to all patients receiving total parenteral nutrition at least twice a week to prevent essential fatty acid deficiency.

(c) Miscellaneous energy sources

Fructose gained popularity as an energy source because it was considered not to be dependent on insulin for its metabolism. However 30% of the infused fructose is converted to lactate and pyruvate and the remainder to glucose which requires insulin for its further metabolism. Furthermore hyperuricaemia and metabolic acidosis have been associated with fructose infusion. Sorbitol is largely converted to fructose.

Xylitol may also lead to a number of adverse effects including nausea, renal impairment and acidosis. Nevertheless xylitol has attracted recent interest as an additional energy source for stressed patients who are dextrose intolerant. Xylitol enters the alternative pathway (described in Section 2.4.2) which generates nucleotides for protein synthesis and intermediates for fat metabolism. Ethanol has a high energy value but organ toxicity such as impaired leukocyte migration, phagocytosis, and function of the respiratory cilia precludes its use.

6.2.2 NITROGEN SOURCE

Many formulations of synthetic crystalline laevo amino acids are now available, and they are more efficiently utilized than protein hydrolysates which have been superseded. Examples of some of these general purpose preparations are given in Table 6.3. Their composition is based on that of high class protein such as egg yolk or human milk.

(a) Amino acids

All preparations contain the essential amino acids which collectively constitute approximately 40% of the total amino acid content. They differ in their amino acid profile and some preparations contain relatively large amounts of glutamate, aspartate, or glycine to achieve the desired total amino acid concentration. Despite early controversy there is no good evidence that the difference in profile of the current preparations in common use is of clinical relevance.

(b) Electrolytes

Differences in the electrolyte content can be important. As shown in Table 6.3, measured differences are found in the sodium, potassium, magnesium, calcium and phosphate concentrations between different solutions. For example the need for additional phosphate must be remembered when changing from Synthamin to Vamin or Aminoplex, especially if Intralipid is not being administered concurrently. Such confusion can be avoided by familiarity with a limited range of solutions.

(c) Nitrogen requirements

Recent studies suggest the provision of 150 kcal/g of nitrogen (0.63 MJ/g of nitrogen) although a lower ratio may be required in severely hypercatabolic patients. Nitrogen provision of 0.2 g per kg is usually satisfactory but this may need increasing to 0.3 g of nitrogen per kg in stressed patients.

Table 6.3 Nitrogen source: some proprietary preparations

Preparation	Nitrogen g/l	K$^+$	Mg^{2+}	Electrolytes mmol/l Na$^+$	Acetate	Cl$^-$	H$_2$PO$_4^-$
Aminoplex 12	12.4	30	2.5	35	5	67	
Aminoplex 14	13.4	30		35		79	
Aminoplex 24	24.9	30	2.5	35	5	67	
Synthamin 9	9.1	60	5	73	100	70	30
*Synthamin 14	14.0	60	5	73	130	70	30
Synthamin 17	16.5	60	5	73	150	70	30
Vamin 9	9.4	20	1.5	50		55	
*Vamin 14	13.5	50	8	100	135	100	

*Available without electrolytes

Assessment of nitrogen loss by analysis of 24 hours urinary urea excretion should be undertaken as an index of potential nitrogen requirement, and is described in Section 6.6. It must be emphasized that the administration of large amounts of nitrogen and energy will not prevent catecholamine mediated gluconeogenesis in septic patients and may impose further metabolic stress. The provision of more than 18 g of nitrogen and 2800 kcal (11.8 MJ) can rarely be justified.

6.2.3 ELECTROLYTES AND TRACE ELEMENTS

Conservation of sodium is efficient in the stable patient and the administration of 1 mmol/kg per day will usually suffice. Frequently requirements are very much greater with additional allowance having to be made for large losses into the gastrointestinal tract, via external fistulae, or through the skin and respiratory tract. When sodium needs fluctuate it may be advisable to administer supplements separately from the compounded solutions for greater flexibility.

The ability to conserve or excrete potassium is not so well developed and may be impaired in the ill patient. Potassium requirements therefore need close monitoring. Potassium facilitates the incorporation of nitrogen into cell protein and intakes of 6 mmol/g of nitrogen are recommended and between 60–120 mmol per day are usually prescribed.

The daily requirements for calcium, magnesium, and phosphorus are met in most patients by the administration of 7–10 mmol, 3 mmol, and 30 mmol respectively. It should be remembered that large amounts of magnesium may be lost through intestinal secretions, so patients with fistulae in Crohn's disease will need additional supplements. Furthermore phosphate is provided in some commercial amino acid solutions.

The administration of trace elements is less important in the short-term and for patients receiving supplemental parenteral nutrition, but supplements should always be given to the malnourished and patients receiving long-term total parenteral nutrition. In practice it is customary to add a trace element solution such as Addamel to the nutrient solution. Two problems exist with the current solutions: firstly they do not offer a complete spectrum of trace elements and secondly no allowance is made for trace elements which are found as contaminants during the manufacture of parenteral nutrition solu-

Table 6.4   Trace elements: those which are essential in man, those contained in Addamel and potential contaminants

Essential in man	Addamel*	Contaminants
Chromium	Copper	Copper
Cobalt	Fluoride	Manganese
Copper	Iodide	Zinc
Iodide	Iron	
Iron	Manganese	
Manganese	Zinc	
Selenium		
Zinc		

*New formulation containing selenium will soon be marketed

Table 6.5   Content of trace element solutions

Element	Addamel	Travenol Electrolyte A
Calcium	5 mmol	13 mmol
Magnesium	1.5 mmol	14 mmol
Chloride	13.3 mmol	54 mmol
Iron	50 μmol	
Zinc	20 μmol	40 μmol
Manganese	40 μmol	20 μmol
Copper	5 μmol	
Fluoride	50 μmol	
Iodide	1 μmol	

tions. Table 6.4 lists the content of Addamel and trace elements currently considered to be important. There is no provision for selenium, but this omission has been rectified in new solutions which will soon be available. Trace element content of two commercial preparations is compared in Table 6.5.

6.2.4 VITAMINS

Water soluble vitamins are provided in commercially compounded solutions, the contents of which are given in Table 6.6. Solivito

Table 6.6 Examples of adult vitamin preparations for parenteral nutrition
(contents of 1 vial)

Vitamin	Multibionta	Solivito	Vitlipid
B1 (Thiamin)	50 mg	1.2 mg	
B2 (Riboflavin)	10 mg	2.5 mg	
B3 (Pantothenic Acid)	25 mg	10 mg	
B6 (Pyridoxine)	15 mg	2 mg	
B12 (Cyanocobalamin)	—	2 μg	
Nicotinic Acid	100 mg	10 mg	
Folic Acid	—	100 μg	
C (Ascorbic Acid)	500 mg	30 mg	
*E (Tocopherol)	5 mg	—	9.1 mg
H (Biotin)	—	300 μg	
A (Retinol)	39.6 mg	—	0.99 mg
K	—	—	150 μg
D (Cholecalciferol)	—	—	5 μg

*E Tocoperol is also supplied in Intralipid
Note. Revised formulation of Solivito containing increased amounts of Vitamin C is
soon to be marketed

includes a broad spectrum of vitamins but there is insufficient ascorbic
acid, thiamin, and folate. However, a new Solivito solution in which
these deficiencies have been corrected will soon be available. Conversely Multibionta contains excess Vitamin A. These solutions are
frequently alternated to improve vitamin supply. Fat soluble vitamins
D, K, and A are provided in Vitlipid which is added to Intralipid. This
addition is not recommended when Intralipid is administered in compounded three litre bags. Intralipid itself contains Vitamin E.

6.2.5 NEWER SUBSTRATES

(a) Nitrogen sources

Branch chain amino acids have a role in the management of portal
systemic encephalopathy in patients with chronic liver disease and this
is discussed in Chapter 7. There have been claims that branch chain
enriched solutions lead to improved nitrogen balance in trauma and
sepsis, but these have not always been substantiated and further
evaluation is required before routine use can be recommended.

The need to provide additional amino acids which are traditionally regarded as non-essential may be considered under certain circumstances in which endogenous production can be inadequate. Glutamine, tyrosine and cystine may be required respectively in catabolic states, uraemia, and childhood. Poor solubility or stability prevent their addition to intravenous preparations and their incorporation into di and tri-peptides is currently under investigation.

(b) Lipids

Other developments under evaluation include the use of synthetic short chain glycerides which are more water soluble and may avoid the need for emulsifiers, and the role of exogenous carnitine in the enhancement of fat utilization. One disadvantage of short chain glycerides is the potential risk of acidosis.

6.3 Nutrient administration

The development of a simple nutrient delivery system has greatly facilitated administration and enhanced the safety of parenteral nutrition.

6.3.1 THE NUTRIENT CONTAINER

(a) The collapsible plastic bag

All nutrients including Intralipid can be compounded in a collapsible plastic bag under sterile conditions in the pharmacy. A typical bag is illustrated in Fig. 6.1. When Intralipid is included certain precautions are required. The bag must be made of ethylene vinyl acetate and not polyvinyl chloride to prevent leaching of plasticizers, and the recommended concentrations of divalent ions must not be exceeded. The addition of excess divalent ions reduces the electrostatic charge on the fat globules which subsequently aggregate. This means that 'all in one' mixes containing Intralipid are unsuitable for use in patients who need additional magnesium or zinc, these ions must be infused separately.

The use of such three litre containers avoids the need for simultaneous infusion from separate bottles. This simplifies treatment, saves nursing time, and reduces the risk of air embolism and infection.

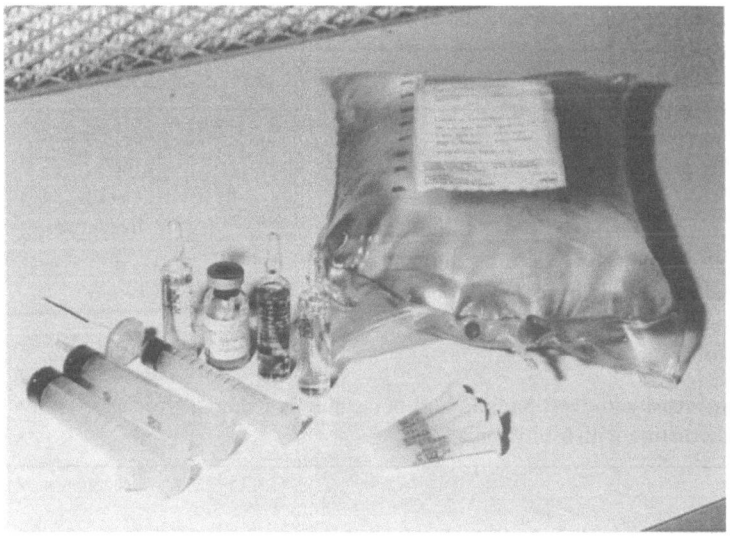

Figure 6.1 Collapsible three-litre bag containing nutrient solutions

Nevertheless in critically ill patients with fluctuating fluid and electrolyte requirements it may still be expedient to administer these components separately.

(b) The bottle system

Smaller hospitals may lack pharmacy facilities for nutrient compounding. Under these circumstances it is customary to attach three parallel lines to the central catheter for the simultaneous infusion from separate bottles of energy (dextrose or lipid), amino acids, and electrolyte solutions. One manufacturer (Giestlich) provides a dextrose electrolyte solutions, Glucoplex, which is designed to be run in parallel with the amino acid solution Aminoplex.

6.3.2 NUTRIENT REGIMES

Following the introduction of the compounded bags it became evident that the majority of patients could be treated satisfactorily with a limited range of regimes. In our hospital three such standard bags are employed, the contents of which are illustrated in Table 6.7.

Table 6.7 Examples of 'standard' parenteral nutrition solutions

Solution	(1)	(2)	(3)
Contents			
Energy (kcal)	2000	2000	1400
	1000 as		1000 as
	Intralipid		Intralipid
Nitrogen (gN)	14	14	10
Additional additives	None	Mg Zn Ca	None
(as required)		Insulin	
Volume	2000	2000	3000

Standard additives: Sodium and potassium as required, Addamel, Solivito alternating with Multibionta

The third regime is designed for infusion into a peripheral vein. This supplies 1400 kcal (6.6 MJ) including 140 g of dextrose and 10 g of nitrogen. The osmolality is less than 600 mosm/l which is the maximum tolerable for peripheral infusion and a third of that found with some of the 'central' regimes.

Obviously these regimes will not satisfy all adult requirements. Severely stressed or burnt patients are provided with solutions which contain 18 g of nitrogen and 2700 kcal (11.3 MJ), 1000 kcal (4.2 MJ) of which are in the form of lipid. Concentrated amino acid sources such as Aminoplex 24 are of particular value in patients who cannot tolerate a volume load.

The clinician responsible for the supervision of patients who need parenteral nutrition must understand their requirements and communicate with the pharmacist. A comprehensive prescription and requisition form is helpful and serves to reduce misunderstanding and nutrient wastage. The prescription form in use in our unit is shown in Fig. 6.2.

6.3.3 NUTRIENT DELIVERY

(a) Route of infusion

(i) Peripheral Provided the patient can tolerate this volume, a peripheral regime will usefully maintain the nutritional status in many

PARENTERAL NUTRITION REQUISITION FORM

see 'Requisition Form - Explanatory Notes'
(a copy should be kept in the ward)

for further information, forms or notes -
contact Area Pharmaceutical Laboratory,
Ninewells Hospital, 2165

PATIENT'S NAME

Unit No		Ward
Hospital		Consultant
Sex	Wt	Ht

DIAGNOSIS:

Why is enteral feeding impossible or inadequate ?

How long is it since dietary intake was normal? . . . . Estimated weight loss. . . . . .Serum albumin . . . . .g/l

Please tick as appropriate -

Mobility.	"Trauma":	Sepsis:	Renal failure:
on IPPV ☐	< 7 days post-op ☐	mild ☐	requiring dialysis ☐
awake in bed ☐	single fracture ☐	moderate ☐	renal failure not requiring dialysis ☐
up to sit ☐	multiple fractures ☐	severe ☐	
up and about ☐	burns ☐ (state total % . . . . .)	severe plus respiratory failure ☐	

is parenteral nutrition to be supplemental ☐ or total ☐ ?

Is the feeding line in situ?   Yes ☐   No ☐

Signature of
CONSULTANT
in charge . . . .

Day	Date	Is a new bag of P.N. Solution required ?	Solution Required	Do the contents of standard solution require to be modified?	Start time	Signature
					Rate	Designation
1		Yes ☐ No ☐	1 ☐ other ☐ ·· please specify ↓ 2 ☐ 3 ☐	No ☐ Yes ☐ ·· specify ↓	ml/24hrs	
2		Yes ☐ No ☐	1 ☐ other ☐ ·· please specify ↓ 2 ☐ 3 ☐	No ☐ Yes ☐ ·· specify ↓	ml/24hrs	
3		Yes ☐ No ☐	1 ☐ other ☐ ·· please specify ↓ 2 ☐ 3 ☐	No ☐ Yes ☐ ·· specify ↓	ml/24hrs	

Figure 6.2 Parenteral nutrition prescription form

patients for short periods. It is easier to supervise and avoids many of the hazards associated with central feeding. However the nutrient content is inadequate for many patients, and it is unsuitable for long periods as it immobilizes the patient.

(ii) Central Nutrient solutions which satisfy the needs of stressed and malnourished patients are too hyperosmolar to infuse peripherally and need to be infused into a central vein through a Silastic catheter. This arrangement is also more suitable for prolonged treatment offering a 'permanent' venous access and allowing increased patient mobility when prolonged treatment is envisaged.

(b) Flow control

The rate of flow requires careful control as the rapid infusion of the contents of a three litre bag may be lethal. Control can be achieved with a flow-limiting device, such as Isoflux (Giestlich), but most clinicians prefer to use a volumetric pump. Many types of pump are currently available. In addition to accuracy and reliability they should not pump air, generate high pressures in the event of catheter occlusion, or allow the back-flow of blood. Warning devices are essential for air-in-line or occlusion, and battery operation in the event of mains failure is also important. The IMED 960 is an example of a well designed pump which is safe and easy to use, particularly for the patient who is receiving treatment at home.

(c) Continuous v. cyclical infusion

Initially nutrients are infused continuously, but in stable patients intermittent or cyclical parenteral nutrition is preferred. The patient infuses overnight and disconnects the giving set from the catheter during the day. Catheter patency is maintained by injecting a solution of heparin in saline through a latex-ended spigot. The techniques involved are discussed later.

Cyclical parenteral nutrition frees the patient during the day, facilitating mobilization and physiotherapy. In all but the most severely ill patients metabolic advantages include reduced water and fat with equivalent nitrogen retention.

6.4 Central venous catheters

The success of parenteral nutrition depends on the careful placement and meticulous management of the central venous catheter. Catheters are placed in the superior vena cava through the subclavian vein or a tributary, and the proximal end is tunnelled subcutaneously to emerge from the anterior chest wall. Particular care must be taken of the exit site and junction with the giving set or spigot to minimize the risk of infection. Neglect of this device is common in departments unaccustomed to central feeding and results in avoidable and potentially serious complications. Catheter associated complications are discussed in Section 6.5.

6.4.1 CATHETER DESIGN

(a) Catheter material

Catheters should be strong, soft and inert to prevent damage to the vessel wall. The majority of catheters are made of silicon, which is less thrombogenic and much softer than polyvinyl chloride, or polyurethane. Recently catheters made of polyurethane have been introduced. This material is as pliable as silicon at body temperatures, and shares a low thrombogenicity but in addition it has a greater tensile strength.

(b) Catheter type

Four types of catheter are in current use. The first has a detachable hub, the second a fixed hub and a teflon cuff, and a third an implantable subcutaneous chamber at its proximal end. The recent introduction of a catheter with a distal valve Groshong (Cath Tech) promises to facilitate management by eliminating clamping and reducing the risk of retrograde blood flow or air embolism.

(i) Catheters with detachable hubs   Two examples of catheters with detachable hubs are shown in Fig. 6.3. The Vygon Neutricath S is a silicon elastomer catheter, the Viggo Secalon Nucath is made of polyurethane and has an 'on/off' switch at the hub. Detachable hubs make insertion and tunnelling easier: this is readily accomplished under local anaesthesia with minimal trauma to the patient. Great care

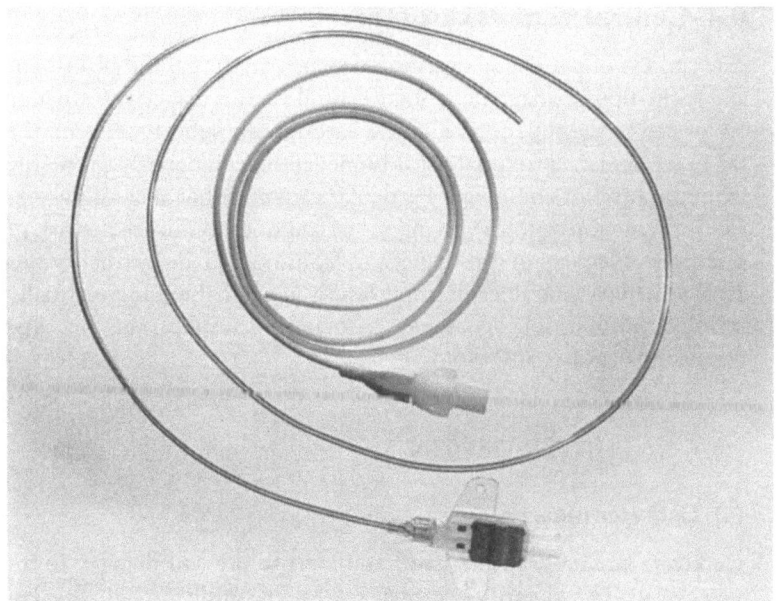

Figure 6.3 Vygon and Viggo catheters with detachable hubs. Note the on/off switch on the hub of the Viggo catheter

must be taken when assembling the hub to avoid subsequent detachment with the risk of catheter embolization. These catheters are anchored by suturing the hub to the skin, a potential source of infection adjacent to the exit site. The switch on the Viggo hub is theoretically attractive, obviating the need to clamp the catheter when changing giving sets. Unfortunately the crevices are difficult to clean, its use may result in tension on the sutures, and the valve mechanism creates a dead space facilitating blood 'flash-back' during cyclical nutrition.

(ii) Cuffed catheters with fixed hubs   The Broviac catheter (Fig. 6.4) is a preferred design for long-term treatment. In addition to the fixed hub there is a teflon cuff which lies in a subcutaneous tunnel and stimulates a fibrotic reaction. Originally this was developed as a barrier against infection spreading down the external surface of the catheter. However its real value is that it serves as an anchor preventing any movement of the catheter in the subcutaneous tunnel and avoiding the need

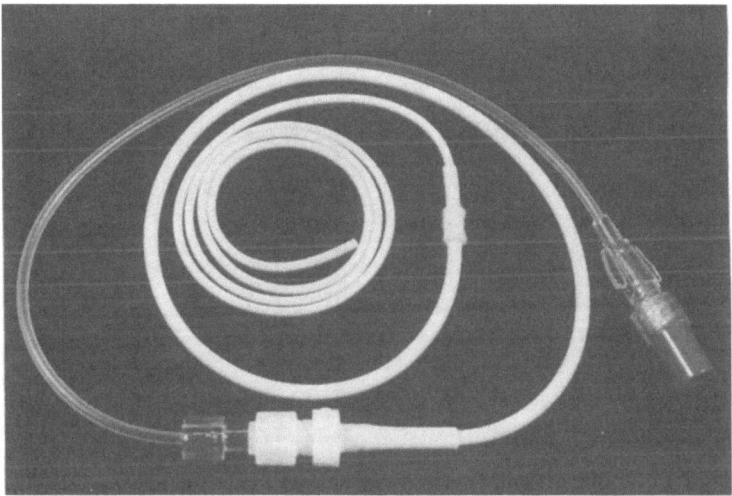

Figure 6.4 The Broviac catheter with a fixed hub and teflon cuff

for external sutures. The Hickman catheter is similar to the Broviac design except for a larger internal diameter (1.8 mm compared with 1.0 mm) which facilitates the administration of blood products. It has no advantage for nutrient supply and is more commonly employed in oncology. Cuffed Vygon catheters have recently become available.

(iii) Implanted catheters For all patients receiving parenteral nutrition, the external catheter poses a threat of infection and for those requiring prolonged treatment it is an inconvenience. In order to facilitate catheter management, reduce the risk of infection, and allow the patient greater freedom, small volume stainless steel injectable ports have been developed which are implanted subcutaneously. An example is the Port-a-Cath (Pharmacia Nu-Tech), shown in Fig. 6.5. The stainless steel chamber is covered by a latex injection port and connected to a silicon rubber catheter. The giving set is attached to a specially designed needle which is placed through the carefully cleaned skin which overlies the injection port. These devices were initially introduced for the administration of intermittent chemo-therapy, but experience of use for nutrient delivery in patients receiving home parenteral nutrition is increasing. They enable the patient to participate in a wider range of activities for example swim-

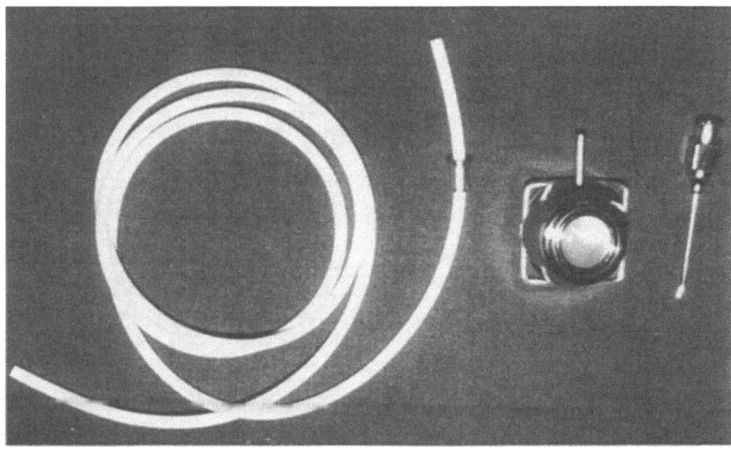

Figure 6.5 The Port-a-Cath system with an implantable stainless steel chamber covered by a latex injection port

ming and they may help reduce the incidence of infection. Some patients find the needle insertion painful and unattractive.

6.4.2 CATHETER INSERTION

This is a full aseptic technique which is best achieved in the operating theatre using image intensification X-ray facilities. It is never an emergency procedure. Meticulous care is required to avoid damage to surrounding structures, introduction of infection, and inappropriate locations. The catheter should lie in the superior vena cava with the tip just above the right atrium. Complications are reviewed in the next sections but they include pneumothorax, damage to the subclavian artery, thoracic duct or brachial plexus, septicaemia, and location in the jugular vein or right ventricle.

(a) Venous access

Insertion may be achieved with a percutaneous Seldinger technique into the infraclavicular subclavian vein. Many authorities prefer the subclavian approach as the exit site is conveniently situated but it is more commonly associated with major complications, and the creation of a subcutaneous tunnel overcomes the problem of exit site location with supraclavicular venous access. The recent introduction of split sheath catheter introducing kits (William Cook, Bloomington Inc.) has improved the safety of such insertions and facilitated the placement of larger Broviac and Hickman catheters. The use of a similar system for the placement of cuffed Vygon catheters is now also available.

The larger catheters are frequently placed by surgical cut-down procedures that avoid the hazard of blind percutaneous puncture. The cephalic external jugular or internal jugular veins are preferred. In exceptional patients with very difficult venous access cannulation of the superior vena cava has been performed using an intercostal tributary of the azygos vein, or catheters have been placed in the right atrium using the atrial appendage at thoracotomy. The inferior vena cava is an unsatisfactory route for prolonged parenteral nutrition. Its use is associated with a high incidence of venous thrombosis and catheters are liable to migrate in the mobile patient.

(b) Skin tunnelling

In the belief that catheter related sepsis gains access from the skin catheter interface at the exit site and tracks down the external surface of the catheter, a subcutaneous tunnel is now employed. The proximal end of the catheter bearing the hub emerges from the skin some 7–10 cm away from the point at which the catheter enters a vein. It is hoped that the tunnel will create a physical barrier and reduce the incidence of catheter related sepsis. It has been claimed that tunnelling delays catheter related sepsis and forewarns of this condition when the exit site becomes reddened. The comparative reduction of incidence with historical control has been taken as evidence of the efficacy of tunnelling for this purpose. However studies have now shown that under strict nursing supervision a tunnel results in no additional reduction of the incidence of sepsis, possibly reflecting the subsequent observation that the exit site is not the major source of infection. Nevertheless a tunnel will reduce this risk when nursing care is sub-optimal and it is useful for two other purposes. It facilitates anchorage of the catheter via the teflon cuff which lies subcutaneously, and it brings the exit site to a more convenient location particularly when the jugular vein has been cannulated. Subcutaneous tunnels are therefore recommended.

(c) Catheter placement

(i) *Infraclavicular approach* After careful skin preparation including shaving where necessary and the application of Povidone-Iodine or similar antiseptic, the patient is covered by sterile drapes and placed in a head-down position to prevent air embolism. Following the infiltration of local anaesthetic, a 1 cm skin incision is made 2 cm below the mid-point of the clavicle. The position of the subclavian vein may be identified using a needle with an attached syringe. The needle is advanced to the inferior aspect of the clavicle and then redirected medially upwards and backwards, angled towards the suprasternal notch and advanced until the subclavian vein is penetrated with a 'flash-back' of venous blood. The needle is withdrawn and the catheter is introduced through the plastic cannula which is then withdrawn. The position of the catheter in the distal superior vena cava is checked and adjusted as necessary. A skin tunnel is created after infiltration with local anaesthetic by an introducer inserted 7–10 cm below the entry point and the proximal end of the catheter without the hub is passed back through the introducer. The hub is attached and the catheter is flushed with heparin and secured by sutures close to its exit site.

Fine bore catheters may be inserted using the Seldinger technique, using either the infraclavicular approach to the subclavian vein or directly into the external jugular vein, and insertion kits are commercially available Centrosyl (Travenol Laboratories) or supplied with the catheter (Vygon). The flexible J-shaped guidewire is advanced through the needle into the superior vena cava. The position of the guidewire is screened and the introducing needle withdrawn. The catheter is then advanced over the guidewire. After adjusting the position the guidewire is withdrawn.

Placement of larger catheters with fixed hub and dacron cuffs, for example Broviac or Vygon Life-Vac, under local anaesthesia has been facilitated by the introduction of split introducers. A skin tunnel is made using a cannula over a needle which is inserted just below the mid-point of the clavicle and directed inferomedially to emerge 10 cm below the entry point on the anterior chest wall. The exit site is enlarged with artery forceps to allow the dacron cuff to pass, the needle is withdrawn, the catheter threaded through the cannula, the position of which is adjusted so that the cuff lies at least 3 cm within the tunnel. The introducing cannula is withdrawn and the free distal end of the catheter is cut to the estimated required length. With the patient in the head-down position the subclavian vein is punctured from the infraclavicular incision using a needle from a cardiac pacemaker lead introduction set (William Cook, Bloomington Inc.). The guidewire is inserted via the needle which is withdrawn and the split sheath introducer is advanced over the guidewire which is also withdrawn. The catheter is passed through the sheath and the two halves of the latter are peeled away as it is withdrawn. The position of the guidewire, introducer and catheter should be screened.

(ii) Surgical exposure techniques These techniques are safer especially for the inexperienced operator. The cephalic vein is conveniently located lying in the delto-pectoral groove. Exposure is achieved via a 3 cm incision, 2 cm below the clavicle in the direction of the groove, with subsequent division of the fascia taking care to avoid the acromio-clavicular artery and lateral pectoral nerves. The vessel is controlled by proximal and distal ligature, and the catheter is tunnelled up to the wound from the exit site and inserted via venotomy. The external jugular vein may be similarly employed just above the clavicle, but the approach to the internal jugular vein is more difficult although it offers good venous access. Catheters of the implantable devices (e.g. Port-a-Cath) may be inserted as previously described and joined to the chamber which is sutured to the underlying fascia. The position of the tunnelled catheter is shown in Fig. 6.6 and the subcutaneous location of the Port-a-Cath in Fig. 6.7.

6.4.3 CATHETER MANAGEMENT

The conscientious observation of a detailed catheter care protocol by experienced nursing staff is essential. Careless catheter management may lead to several serious complications which are poorly tolerated in malnourished patients. Catheter fracture, occlusion, sepsis and air embolism must be avoided.

(a) Extension set

Disconnecting the giving set to change the feed bag or apply a heparin lock is associated with the risk of air embolism. This can be prevented in two ways. The use of the head-down position is not advised as blood 'flash-back' may eventually lead to catheter occlusion, so

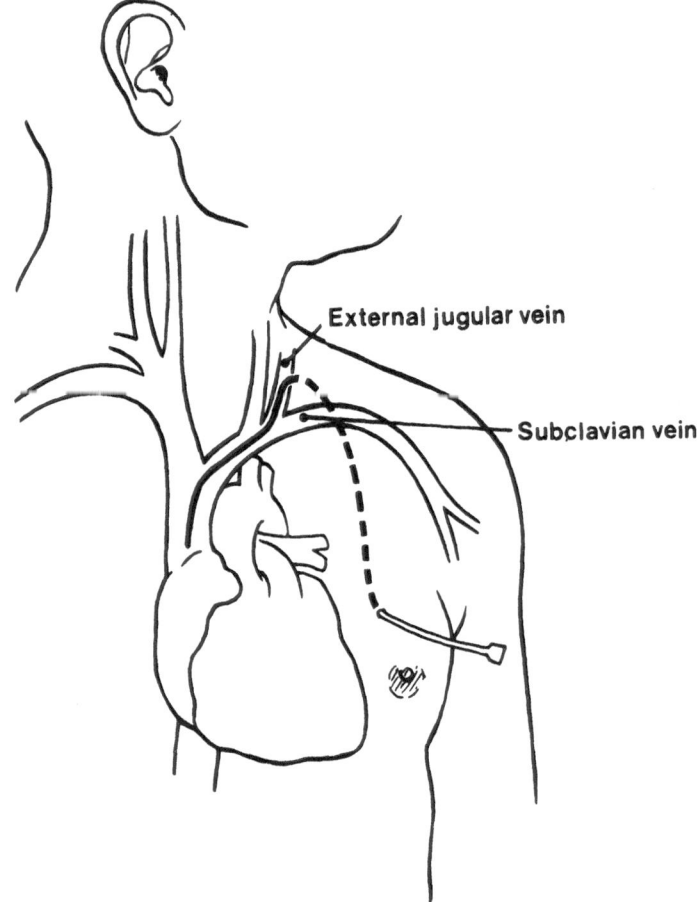

Figure 6.6 The position of the tunnelled catheter

clamping is the method of choice. With prolonged use repeated clamping may damage the catheter and when the need for such treatment is envisaged an extension set (e.g. Lectroflex) between the catheter and giving set is advisible. The extension set is used for clamping. It reduces the movement at the exit site and ensures that the junction with the giving set is more conveniently situated for management by the patient which is important in the home situation. It should be changed every 2–4 weeks. A new generation of catheters

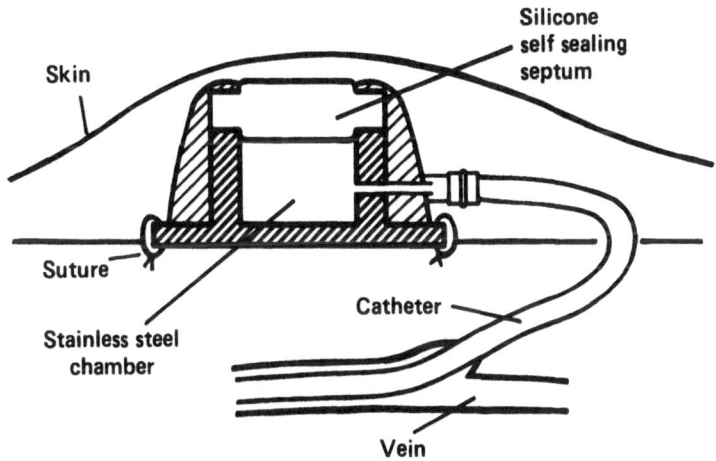

Figure 6.7 The subcutaneous location of the Port-a-Cath

with distal valves may obviate the need for clamping and thus the extension set.

(b) Catheter procedures

Procedures such as changing the giving set, disconnecting the infusion and applying a heparin lock, recommencing infusion, and changing the extension set, must be undertaken using an aseptic technique with sterile gloves and mask. The junctions between the catheter and extension piece, extension piece and giving set or spigot, are bound in sterile swabs impregnated with Betadine. The hub is a major potential source of sepsis.

When the feed bag is changed the protective dressings around the junction between the giving set and catheter or extension set are removed using a no-touch technique. A new sterile Betadine soaked swab is then placed around the junction. Using two other similar swabs the old giving set and distal extension set are wiped away from the junction for a few centimetres in each direction and left for a few minutes. The junction swab is removed, the extension set is clamped and the giving sets exchanged. The junction is once more bound in a Betadine swab. The application of a heparin lock involves similar precautions but instead of the giving set, a sterile latex-ended spigot

(Vygon 891) is applied to the distal end of the extension piece. A saline flush followed by heparin is injected through the spigot, thus avoiding any 'flash-back' which might occur following the release of clamps with conventional plastic spigots.

(c) Exit site

For the first day after catheter insertion the exit site and surrounding skin are covered with Betadine and a sterile gauze dressing. Thereafter a semi-permeable adhesive dressing (Primapore) is applied and changed weekly or more frequently if necessary. The exit site is carefully inspected for any tenderness, redness or exudation which may signify infection.

(d) Alternatives to central venous catheters

Arterio-venous shunts have been employed for the long-term delivery of parenteral nutrition solutions. In spite of anticoagulation which may not be acceptable in many patients, particularly those with inflammatory bowel disease, thrombosis remains a major problem with this procedure.

6.5 Complications of parenteral nutrition

With careful patient selection and management parenteral nutrition is relatively safe but serious potential hazards exist. Many of these can be avoided using peripheral supplemental parenteral nutrition whenever possible. The complications associated with conventional central parenteral nutrition may be conveniently considered in three groups: catheter related complications, metabolic complications and miscellaneous problems.

6.5.1 CATHETER RELATED COMPLICATIONS

A variety of complications may occur during catheter insertion and some are shown in Table 6.8. Examples of the more common catheter related problems which develop during the course of parenteral nutrition are shown in Table 6.9.

Table 6.8   Complications of catheter insertion

Arterial puncture e.g. subclavian artery, carotid artery
Pleural and mediastinal injury e.g. pneumothorax, haemomediastinum
Lymphatic injury e.g. thoracic ducts, laceration
Neurological injury e.g. damage to phrenic nerve, brachial plexus
Embolism: catheter or air
Malposition e.g. internal jugular vein or ventricular

Table 6.9   Catheter related complications

Infection
Thrombosis
Occlusion
Breakage
Air embolism

(a) Mechanical complications during insertion

Most complications involve damage to adjacent structures. These occur less frequently with experienced operators and when subclavicular insertion is avoided. Air embolism is prevented by using the head-down position, and great care must be taken to ensure the catheter does not embolize, particularly when using catheters with detachable hubs. Occasionally catheters pass into the internal jugular veins or lie too distally in the right ventricle. Use of catheters in such positions may respectively cause cerebral thrombophlebitis or cardiac dysrhythmia and even cardiac tamponade as the catheter tip is prone to lodge and eventually move through the right ventricular wall. Screening the catheter position during and following insertion is essential.

(b) Catheter related infection

This is one of the most frequently reported complications. The wide range of incidence reported in the early literature reflects differences in patients groups, diagnostic criteria, catheter care procedures, and the purpose for which catheters were used. Given appropriate care, the incidence of serious catheter related infection should be very low, in

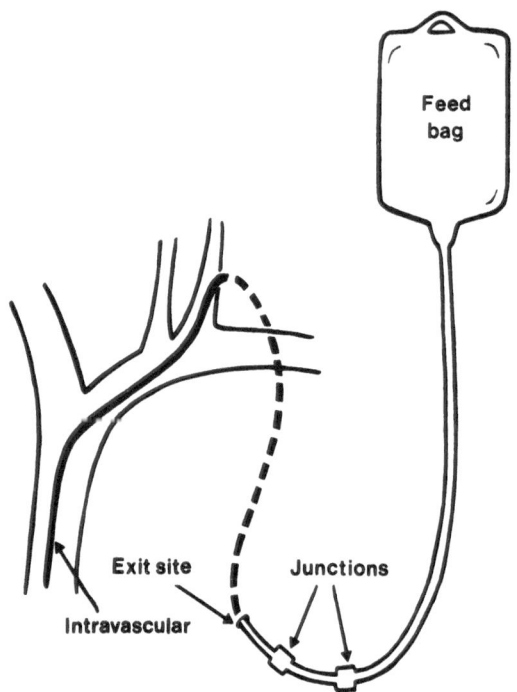

Figure 6.8 Catheter-related sepsis: routes of infection

our own experience less than 1% or one per ten patient years of hospital treatment.

(i) Definition Catheter related infection can take two forms. First a simple exit site infection with tenderness, reddening and exudation from the catheter skin interface. Second and more seriously a bacter-aemia in the absence of an obvious primary source when the same organism is cultured from the catheter and blood. In the latter situation the exit site usually appears uninfected.

(ii) Source of infection Catheters may become infected by four routes which are shown in Fig. 6.8. Very few examples of contamination of the nutrient solution have been reported, though clearly all catheters may become colonized by haematogenous spread. Traditional thinking supports the view that micro-organisms spread down the external catheter surface from the exit site: the subcutaneous tunnel

and the dacron cuff were both conceived as barriers to this process. However the reported association between microbial growth on the skin at the exit site and the subsequent development of catheter related infection has been criticized because of failure to identify the species of micro-organism. It has been claimed that bacteria responsible for catheter infections differ from those cultured at the exit site.

More recently elegant prospective studies have demonstrated that catheter hub colonization is the most frequent source of catheter related sepsis, leading to progressive intraluminal colonization. Furthermore many catheters are colonized by micro-organisms without clinical evidence of infection. This particularly applies to coagulase-negative Staphylococci which readily adhere to catheter materials and become surrounded by a mucilaginous slime. The probability of associated catheter related septicaemia is related to the density of colonization, and a density equal to or less than 15 colonies on the plate distinguishes colonization from infection.

(iii) The nature of infecting micro-organisms The organisms most commonly responsible for catheter related septicaemia in patients receiving parenteral nutrition are Staphylococcus epidermis, Staphylococcus aureus, Escherichia coli and Candida species. The spectrum is much wider in patients who are immunosuppressed, particularly those with neoplastic disease.

(iv) Diagnosis The diagnosis of exit site infection is straightforward. Catheter related septicaemia is signified by the development of pyrexia and tachycardia. Unfortunately many patients who require parenteral nutrition have other causes for these features including sepsis in the post-operative patient and active Crohn's disease. Resolution of the temperature and tachycardia following removal of the catheter is the ultimate diagnostic confirmation but such an approach would lead to the unnecessary removal of many catheters.

The presence of a pathogen such as Staphylococcus epidermis in blood cultures is strongly suggestive of catheter related sepsis. In most centres several peripheral and catheter blood cultures for bacteria and fungi are obtained on suspicion of catheter sepsis. Central blood cultures have the theoretical disadvantage of risking catheter thrombosis and internal catheter contamination in the presence of unrelated bacteraemia. The need for central cultures has recently been disputed but they should always be obtained in immunocompromised patients.

Routine culture of the removed catheter tip may give a false positive result unless a semi-quantitative method is used to distinguish colonization from infection, as more infections are associated with a confluent growth. This principle has been extended to the use of gram staining of removed catheter segments, providing a rapid diagnosis with views of both the external and internal catheter surfaces.

(v) Prevention of catheter related infection   Catheter related infection is largely avoidable using the methods described. These obviate the need for proposed measures such as the use of low dose heparin infusion, in-line filters (although these may be of value for other reasons), or the addition of a non-toxic antimicrobial Taurolin to the nutrient solution. The need for prophylactic antibiotics to cover invasive procedures or dental extractions should be considered in an attempt to prevent colonization.

(vi) Treatment of suspected catheter related infection   When a patient who is receiving parenteral nutrition develops a temperature and a tachycardia, it is essential first to try and exclude other sources of infection by careful examination and preliminary investigation. This includes urine microscopy, chest X-ray, blood and possibly catheter cultures. Thereafter three options should be considered:

- Removal of the catheter
- Removal of the catheter and provision of broad spectrum anti-microbial cover to include Staphylococcus epidermis and Staphylococcus aureus
- Leaving the catheter in position and prescribing antibiotics pending the results of preliminary blood cultures

These decisions will depend upon the availability and importance of venous access, the patient's immune competence and the need for continuation of treatment.

In the event of continuing symptoms after catheter withdrawal or negative cultures, other reasons for the illness should be sought. Conversely positive cultures especially with Staphylococci are suggestive of catheter related sepsis. If the catheter is still in position, there are again three options. These are:

- Removal
- Exchange over guidewire (which will inevitably lead to the contamination of a proportion of replaced catheters)

● Attempts to eradicate the infection by antimicrobial chemo-therapy administered through the catheter

In addition to antibiotics some clinicians have advocated the application of locks of solutions containing hydrochloric acid or 70% ethanol, but the value and safety of such substances have not been substantiated. Antibiotic therapy may be successful in the resolution of catheter related sepsis, but the risk of superior vena cava thrombosis and metastatic infection, such as osteomyelitis, must not be overlooked. Attempts to manage patients in this way should be reserved for those dependent on treatment in whom venous access is very difficult. A urokinase lock may enhance antimicrobial penetration by reducing the fibrin sheath around the catheter tip.

(c) Venous thrombosis

(i) Pathogenesis Following insertion, catheters become incased in a fibrin sheath which starts within 24 hours from the point of entry into the vein and where the catheter tip touches the vessel wall. It propagates to involve the entire catheter within 1–2 weeks. This is one of the factors which may be implicated in thrombus formation. Others include catheter infection, osmolality and duration of treatment, although not all studies have confirmed their role.

Autopsy studies of high risk patients report thrombosis in over 50%, whereas studies using prospective venography have demonstrated thrombus in 20–50% of patients. The majority of such thrombi are occult, and clinical evidence of venous occlusion is apparent in any 0.2 to 4.8% of patients.

It is important to note that the propensity to venous thrombosis is related to catheter material. Silicon is much less thrombogenic than polyvinyl chloride although even with silicon thrombosis may be as high as 40% when sought prospectively. Polyurethane is also thought to have a lower thrombogenicity similar to that of silicon rubber.

(ii) Clinical features The development of pyrexia in the absence of infection, unexplained tachycardia or pain in the chest or at the root of the neck, are features which prompt the search for venous thrombosis by phlebography before venous occlusion becomes apparent. Failure to recognize these features and persistence with treatment will invariably lead to evidence of subclavian or superior vena cava thrombosis and pulmonary emboli may ensue.

(iii) Prevention   The risk of venous thrombosis can be reduced by employing Silastic or polyurethane catheters. The use of heparin infused in a dose of 5000 units 6 hourly has been shown to lower the incidence of thrombosis in prospective venographic studies. Unfortunately this is not practical for many post-operative patients and leads to the development of osteoporosis during long-term treatment. Because clinically significant thrombosis and embolization are uncommon, heparin is not advised for routine use but may be reserved for high risk patients.

(iv) Management   Established venous thrombosis necessitates the temporary cessation of central venous feeding, but peripheral feeding may be used to tide the patient over if necessary. The clinician is required to make two decisions, whether to remove the catheter or leave it in position, and whether to treat the patient with Streptokinase followed by heparin or heparin alone.

If the patient is not severely ill and continued central parenteral nutrition is not considered to be essential, a heparin infusion should be established and the catheter withdrawn after 2–3 days. Conversely in the presence of severe acute superior vana cava occlusion or if continued central nutrition is essential a Streptokinase infusion is given for 24 hours followed by heparin. Careful haematological monitoring is necessary and sequential phlebography is used to monitor the resolution of the thrombus.

(d) Catheter occlusion

Catheters may block due to thrombus, lipid deposits, or amorphous debris.

(i) Thrombotic occlusion   Thrombotic occlusion may follow blood 'flash-back' which occurs when connections leak, with faulty catheter techniques, or in association with a gradual build-up of fibrin around the tip of the catheter. If recognized, the instillation of a solution of Urokinase (5000 units in 3 ml of saline for 3 hours) into a partially blocked catheter may clear the occlusion. This will not clear catheters which have blocked for other reasons.

(ii) Lipid occlusion   Following the introduction of lipid containing 'all in one' mixes several reports have described the deposition of

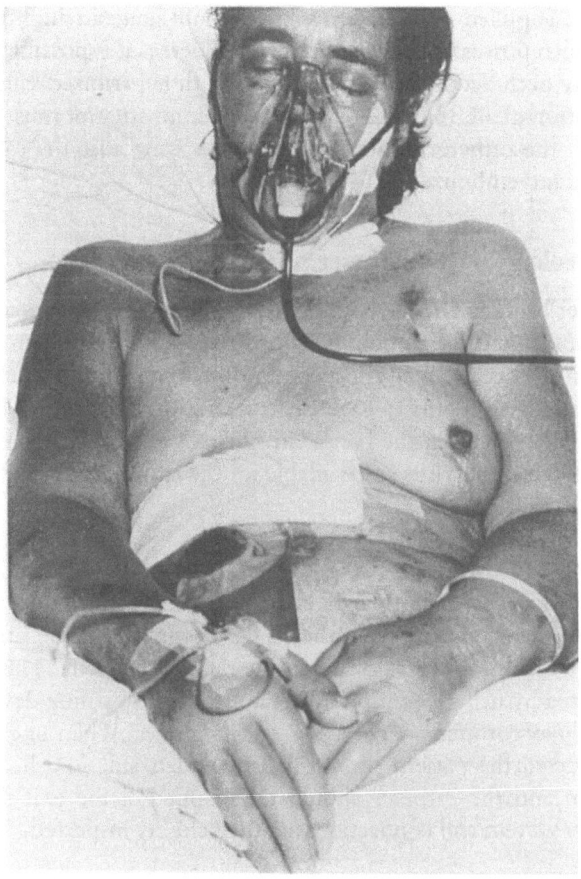

Figure 6.9 Facial and upper limb oedema following thrombosis of the superior vena cava

lipid-like material in the catheter lumen which was not previously observed when Intralipid was infused separately. The lipid deposit may be avoided by a separate lipid infusion or by adding no divalent ions to lipid containing bags. This phenomena is only observed during prolonged treatment as is occlusion due to amorphous crystalline material. Lipid deposits may be removed by the instillation of a 50% ethanol solution which is left in the catheter for one hour before flushing and heparinization.

Because of the occasional occurrence of catheter occlusion patients must be supplied with pumps which do not generate high pressures and which possess an occlusion alarm. Whereas it is possible to free a partially occluded catheter by flushing with heparinized saline or the application of a Urokinase or ethanol lock, no attempt must be made to flush the catheter under pressure. This can cause the catheter to rupture and embolize.

(e) Breakage of the catheter

Catheter breakage occurred more commonly before the provision of extension sets for clamping and may follow aggressive attempts to clear an occlusion. Daily inspection of the hub during the catheter procedure is advisable to look for cracking. In the event of breakage the catheter between the break and the exit site should be clamped. Commercial repair kits are available for the larger cuffed catheters.

(f) Air embolism

Air embolism is not only a danger during catheter insertion it may also occur as a result of a broken catheter, faulty connection, unsatisfactory catheter care procedures or air in the delivery system. The latter is prevented by using a pump with an appropriate warning device. The patient may complain of chest pain and dyspnoea. When air embolism is suspected the patient should lie on the left side in a head-down position and the catheter should be clamped at the exit site. The delivery system and connections are then closely inspected.

6.5.2 METABOLIC COMPLICATIONS

Metabolic complications are listed in Table 6.10. They may be considered in two groups.

(a) Short-term complications

(i) *Abnormalities of glucose haemostasis*   Patients who harbour sepsis or who are traumatized or burnt are resistant to insulin for which catecholamne and cortisol release are in part responsible. Under these circumstances additional insulin may be needed to prevent hyper-glycaemia with the attendant risk of impaired immune function and hyperosmolar dehydration. If the patient's requirements are stable the

Table 6.10   Metabolic complications

Short-term
Impaired fluid balance
Electrolyte imbalance
Disturbance of pH
Disturbed glucose homeostasis
Increased CO_2 production

Long term
Abnormal liver function tests
Cholelithiasis
Micronutrient deficiency
Metabolic bone disease

addition of insulin to the nutrient bag may be satisfactory, and in spite of adherence to the plastic container 1 unit per 10 g of dextrose is sufficient. For many patients the separate subcutaneous administration of all or part of their insulin needs gives better flexibility of management.

The reverse problem of hypoglycaemia develops transiently when the infusion is suddenly stopped. This is particularly likely to occur when all the energy is supplied as dextrose and insulin supplements are needed. Patients receiving home parenteral nutrition must be warned of these dangers. They are reduced by providing some of the energy as lipid and slowing the infusion rate before disconnecting the giving set. Dangerous hypoglycaemia has been described after discontinuing dextrose solutions during the course of haemodialysis.

(ii) Fluid and electrolyte balance   Abnormalities of hydration and serum electrolytes should be corrected before the initiation of parenteral nutrition. Malnourished patient are prone to sodium and water retention early in their treatment, conversely allowance has to be made for additional losses such as occur through enterocutaneous fistulae. Whereas a limited number of standard prescriptions may meet the energy and nitrogen needs of the majority of patients, fluid and electrolytes must be prescribed according to individual requirements. Where these fluctuate the separate peripheral infusion of electrolytes may be helpful. Careful monitoring, discussed in the next section, is essential at the onset of treatment and in the unstable

patient. Caution must be exercised to avoid hyper or hypokalaemia, hypomagnesaemia, and hypophosphataemia. The latter can occur when changing nitrogen sources from solutions such as Synthamin which contain phosphate to Aminoplex or Vamin with no added phosphate. Such a deficiency is associated with tissue hypoxia and may induce neurological features including impaired consciousness. These deficiencies are discussed in more detail in Chapter 4.

(iii) Metabolic acidosis   Metabolic acidosis occurs less frequently now that fructose and ethanol are no longer used for the supply or energy, when they were responsible for excessive lactate production.

(iv) Dextrose intolerance   The provision of excess dextrose leads to steatosis and increased generation of carbon dioxide, a subject which has been discussed earlier in this chapter. The consequent increased ventilatory needs may pose difficulties when patients are being weaned from artifical ventilation.

(b) Long-term complications

(i) Hepatobiliary disease   Abnormalities in liver function tests are often associated with the use of parenteral nutrition. Alkaline phosphatase and gamma glutamyl transpeptidase values are initially increased, sometimes within the first week of treatment, they level out after two to three weeks and thereafter may remain elevated for the duration of treatment. Such changes may be attributable to significant hepatic steatosis with moderate hepatomegaly. This is usually a feature of excessive dextrose administration and the problem may be resolved by supplying part of the energy needs with Intralipid. Occasionally patients develop jaundice and this has been reported to respond to the oral administration of Metronidazole. Metabolites of anaerobic organisms in the intestinal tract have been implicated in this condition.

The development of jaundice or other features of cholestasis prompts the search for cholelithiasis. There is now little doubt that prolonged parenteral nutrition favours the formation of gall stones and acalculus cholecystitis, since as many as 50% of patients form gall bladder sludge after six weeks. Gall bladder stasis would appear to be a major factor in patients who are receiving total as opposed to supplemental parenteral nutrition and thus no food by mouth. Changes in the lithogenic index may also play a part.

Many patients who require parenteral feeding are at risk of hepatic and biliary tract disorders in association with their primary disease. The development of abnormal liver function tests requires careful consideration and evaluation, at least with ultrasonography.

(ii) Micronutrient deficiency   Micronutrient requirements and the consequences of deficiency are discussed in Chapters 3 and 4. The administration of micronutrients is reviewed earlier in this chapter. The importance of ensuring an adequate supply of trace elements and vitamins merits emphasis. This especially applies to patients who require prolonged total parenteral feeding.

(iii) Metabolic bone disease   The failure to provide Vitamin D will lead to osteomalacia. Paradoxically osteomalacia has also been described in conjunction with hypercalcaemia and hypercalciuria in patients receiving long-term treatment with adequate Vitamin D replacement. Withdrawal of Vitamin D in these patients leads to the resolution of their disease.

Cyclical parenteral nutrition has been associated with a negative calcium balance and osteoporosis. The reason for this is not clear but it may relate to the increased buffering requirements associated with the shorter duration of infusion.

6.5.3 GENERAL COMPLICATIONS

(a) Atrophy of the intestinal mucosa

When patients are fed parenterally and receive no enteral nutrition the intestinal mucosa atrophies making the eventual transfer to enteral feeding more difficult. Enteral feeding not only prevents mucosal atrophy, but facilitates intestinal adaption in patients with the short bowel syndrome. For this reason as well as the desirability of reducing gall bladder sludge and containing costs the enteral route should be employed where possible.

(b) The imposition of treatment

The use of parenteral feeding is seen by some patients and staff as a restrictive imposition. Patient mobility and rehabilitation are encouraged when cyclical nutrition is used. For the patient at home consideration should be given to the use of implantable venous access devices. These are cosmetically more acceptable and patients are able to participate more readily in sports such as swimming.

(c) Psychosocial problems

Some patients resent this form of treatment. Their apparent dependence and in some instances inability to cope with all the psychosocial implications are contributory factors. Anxieties about potential complications should be allayed by competent and sympathetic staff, but financial concerns are particularly pressing for patients who do not benefit from a comprehensive Health Service. This treatment is very expensive and in the USA private insurance and public programmes such as Medicare and Medicade cover only 80% of the total cost. The costs are considered in a later section.

Treatment is accepted readily by the majority of patients who have suffered prolonged malnutrition to whom its benefit is obvious. Those people who lose their intestinal function suddenly following a mesenteric vascular catastrophe take longer to adjust.

6.6 Patient monitoring

Careful patient monitoring is essential to define nutrient needs, to assess the effect of treatment, to adapt to changing requirements, and to provide an early warning of impending complications.

Initially the patient's needs may be assessed on the basis of weight, anthropometric measurements, biochemical indices and nature of the illness. The use of these indices is discussed in Chapter 4. Careful biochemical monitoring avoids the development of metabolic complications and clinical assessment allows the early detection or prevention of other complications such as fluid and electrolyte imbalance.

The frequency and nature of monitoring will depend upon the clinical situation. Frequent comprehensive monitoring is essential after the initiation of therapy and in critically ill patients. Stable patients undergoing treatment at home need only be seen every 4–6 weeks. Table 6.11 outlines the basic monitoring protocol, but additional measurements may be helpful in particular patients where facilities exist, for example direct calorimetry to indicate the amount and nature of energy requirements. Some protocols include the

Table 6.11 Suggested monitoring protocol

		Frequency	
Category	Measurement	Acute/hospital	Chronic/home
Clinical	Pulse, BP	4 Hourly	As clinically indicated
	Temp, Respiration	Daily	As clinically indicated
	Fluid balance	Daily	Monthly
	Weight	Daily	Weekly
	Inspection of exit site,	Daily	Daily
	Catheter hub		
Blood	Sodium, potassium chloride, urea, glucose haemoglobin, WCC WCC + lymphocyte count	Daily	Monthly or as clinically indicated
	Calcium, magnesium phosphorus, zinc albumin, transferrin bilirubin, alk. phos. AST, YGTP	Twice weekly	Monthly or as clinically indicated
	Trace elements screen	Not needed in short-term unless malnourished	1–3 Monthly
Urine	Glucose	Daily	Daily
	Volume	Daily	As indicated
	Urea	Daily	As indicated
	Electrolytes	As indicated	As indicated
Anthropometrics	Weight Skin fold thickness Mean arm muscle Circumference	Weekly	Monthly

measurement of delayed hypersensitivity using skin tests to tuberculin and Candida, but this is not of established value.

6.7 Home parenteral nutrition

Major developments and refinements in the technique of parenteral nutrition have occurred during the last decade. The use of single plastic nutrient containers, improvements in venous access and catheter design, and the adoption of strict catheter care protocols are among the most important and have contributed to the enhanced safety and ease with which parenteral nutrition may be applied. This has led to the increased use of home treatment.

Home parenteral nutrition was first introduced in the USA in the early 1970s. It was a more recent development in the United Kingdom where Professor Irving's group in Manchester has established a register of patients receiving treatment at home. This has provided important information on the application and value of home treatment.

6.7.1 INDICATIONS

The reasons for home parenteral nutrition are outlined in Table 6.12.

(a) Crohn's Disease

Crohn's disease is undoubtedly the commonest indication. It may be responsible for diffuse disease, short bowel syndrome, enterocutaneous fistulae and growth retardation, Such patients derive great benefit from treatment which can improve their quality of life dramatically. Fig 6.10 shows the growth chart of one of our patients. At the onset of treatment he was 19 years and 6 months old, prepubertal with the height of an average 11 year old. This shows that latent growth potential can be achieved even when the patient's age is outside the normally accepted limits for growth.

(b) Motility disorders

Patients with scleroderma fare less well, principally because of disease affecting other organ systems. Furthermore, they frequently lack the manual dexterity required to manage the catheter and so become

Table 6.12 Reasons for home parenteral nutrition

Chronic intestinal failure
　Diffuse intestinal disease
　　Crohn's, radiation enteritis

　Motility disorders
　　Scleroderma, idiopathic intestinal pseudo-obstruction
　Short bowel syndrome
　　Crohn's, volvulus, mesenteric vascular disease

Chronic electrolyte imbalance
　High jejunostomy syndrome
　Enterocutaneous fistulae

Miscellaneous
　Neoplasia
　Growth failure

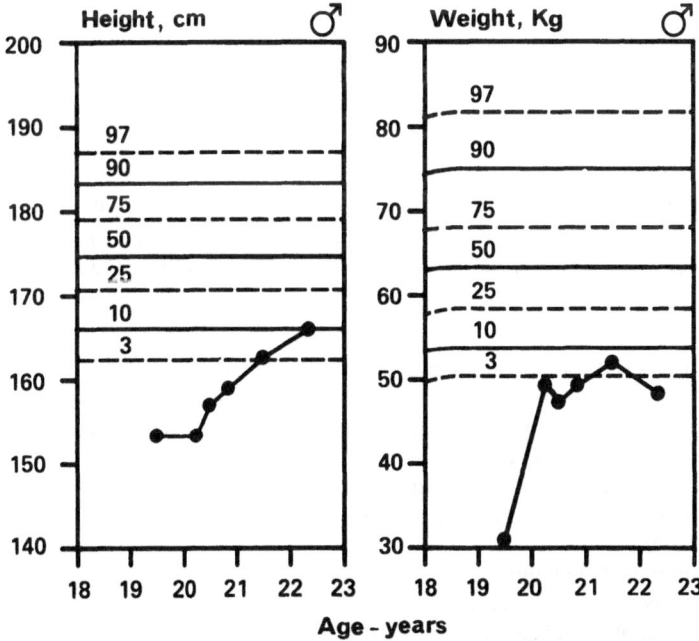

Figure 6.10 Growth and development in a 19-year-old patient with Crohn's disease treated by home parenteral nutrition (Reproduced with permission of the Editor, *British Journal of Hospital Medicine*.)

dependent. Conversely patients with idiopathic intestinal pseudo-obstruction derive much benefit from treatment.

(c) Mesenteric vascular disease

Mesenteric vascular disease may be successfully managed when resection has been undertaken on account of venous thrombosis, such as may follow the use of the oral contraceptive. Patients with arterial disease fare less well, often because of disease affecting other organ systems.

(d) Neoplastic disease

Neoplastic disease in general has been a common reason for home treatment in the USA. The role of parenteral nutrition in the management of neoplastic disease is contentious and relatively few patients have received home treatment for this reason in the United Kingdom.

6.7.2 METHODS

Patients receive cyclical parenteral nutrition as previously described. Before being discharged from hospital they must be carefully trained in catheter management. Their education includes an appreciation of potential complications, their recognition and management. Where possible relatives are involved in this programme. Each patient is supplied with a booklet of procedures, the contents of which are

Table 6.13 Procedure for home parenteral nutrition

Procedure for changing the parenteral feed bag or commencing infusion
Procedure for heparinizing the central line
Procedure for interval heparinization
Procedure for changing the extension piece
Care of the exit site
Use of the IMED pump
Contents of changing packs
Home supplies for parenteral nutrition
Potential problems and management
Emergency procedure for broken catheter

---

shown in Table 6.13. In addition to nutrient bags patients must regularly receive items necessary for catheter care. These include sterile gloves, dressing packs, antiseptic solutions, saline and heparin syringes, spigots and extension sets.

Whilst in hospital, the District Nurse is introduced to the patient and involved in their management. The availability of a refrigerator, telephone and storage space for equipment is checked. After discharge a domiciliary visit to check catheter procedures is advisable.

Home treatment may totally transform the life of recipients who may be relieved of gastrointestinal symptoms, malnutrition, and the need for frequent hospital admissions. Because it is expensive and potentially hazardous, careful selection and supervision is important.

6.8 The cost of parenteral nutrition

The costs incurred by parenteral nutrition are outlined in Table 6.14. This does not take account of the cost of transporting nutrients and other materials and supplying items of equipment such as infusion pumps. Such expenditure can be justified by the immense benefit derived by the patients and their families as well as the reduction in hospital admissions, the ability to work or look after their family, and reduced demands on social services. In some centres costs have been reduced by the local formulation of amino acid solutions and by

Table 6.14 Cost of parenteral nutrition: based on standard two litre bag (see Table 6.7)

	Non-lipid	Lipid bag
	£	£
Nutrients	60.24	71.85
Supplies	1.41	1.41
Labour	1.68	1.68
Equipment for catheter care	5.10	5.10
Total	68.43	80.04

Notes 1) Excludes transport costs for home patients
2) The costs of nutrients are often substantially reduced by discounts available from drug companies

162   Parenteral nutrition

requiring the patients to compound their own nutrient mixtures. Cost must be contained by avoiding excessive nutrient administration and by careful patient selection.

References

Askanazi, J., Carpentier, Y. A., Elwyn, D. H., Nordenström, J., Jeevanandam, M., Rosenbaum, S. H., Gump, F. E. and Kinney, J. M. (1980) The influence of total parenteral nutrition on fuel utilization in injury and sepsis. *Annals of Surgery*, **191**, 40–6.

Black, C. D. and Popovich, N. G. (1981) A study of intravenous emulsion compatibility. Effects of dextrose, amino acids and selected electrolytes. *Drug Intelligence and Clinical Pharmacology*, **15**, 184–8.

Bozetti, F., Scarpa, D., Terno, G., Scotti, A., Ammatuna, M., Bonalumi, M. J. M. and Ceglia, E. (1983) Subclavian venous thrombosis due to indwelling catheters. A prospective study of 52 patients. *Journal of Parenteral and Enteral Nutrition*, **7**, 560–2.

Bozetti, F., Terne, G. and Bonfanti, G. (1984) Blood culture as a guide for the diagnosis of central venous catheter sepsis. *Journal of Parenteral and Enteral Nutrition*, **8**, 396–8.

Burke, J. L., Wolfe, R. R., Mullany, C. J., Mathews, D. E. and Bier, D. M. (1979) Glucose requirements during burn injury. Parameters of optimal glucose infusion and possible hepatic and respiratory abnormalities following excessive glucose intake. *Annals of Surgery*, **190**, 274–85.

Cooper, G. L. and Hopkins, C. C. (1985) Rapid diagnosis of intravascular catheter associated infection by direct gram staining of catheter segments. *New England Journal of Medicine*, **312**, 1142–7.

Elia, M. (1982) The effects of nitrogen and energy intake on the metabolism of normal, depleted and injured man. Considerations for practical nutritional support. *Clinical Nutrition*, **1**, 173–92.

Engels, L. G. J., Skotnichi, S. H. and Burskens, F. G. M. (1983) Home parenteral nutrition via arteriovenous fistulae. *Journal of Parenteral and Enteral Nutrition*, **7**, 412–4.

Fürst, P. (1985) Peptides in parenteral nutrition. *Clinical Nutrition, Special Supplement*, **4**, 105–55.

Gazitua, R., Wilson, K., Bistrian, B. R. and Blackburn, G. (1979) Factors determining peripheral vein tolerance to amino acid infusions. *Archives of Surgery*, **14**, 897–901.

Glynn, M. F. X., Langer, B. and Jeejeebhoy, K. N. (1980) Therapy for thrombotic occlusion of long-term intravenous alimentation catheters. *Journal of Parenteral and Enteral Nutrition*, **4**, 387–90.

Golden, N. H. N. and Golden, B. E. (1981) Trace elements, potential importance in human nutrition with particular reference to zinc and vanadium. *British Medical Bulletin*, **37**, 31–6.

Hoshal, V. L., Ause, R. G., Hoskins, P. A. and Arbor, A. (1971) Fibrin sleeve formation on indwelling subclavian central venous catheters. *Archives of Surgery*, **102**, 353–8.

Jeppsson, K. N., Anderson, G. H., Nakhoods, A. F., Greenberg, G. R., Sanderson, I. and Marliss, E. B. (1976). Metabolic studies in total parental nutrition with lipid in man. *Journal of Clinical Investigation*, **57**, 125–36.

Keohane, P. P., Jones, B. J. M., Attrill, H., Cribb, A., Northover, J., Frost, P. and Silk, D. B. A. (1983) Effect of catheter tunnelling and a nutrition nurse on catheter sepsis during parenteral nutrition. A controlled trial. *Lancet*, **ii**, 1388–90.

Linares, J., Sitges-Serra, A., Garass, J., Percz, J. L. and Martin, R. (1985) Pathogenesis of catheter sepsis: a prospective study with quantitative and semi-quantitative culture of hub and segments. *Journal of Clinical Microbiology*, **21**, 357–60.

MacFie, J., Smith, R. C. and Hill, G. L. (1981) Glucose or fat as a non-protein energy source? A controlled trial in gastroenterological patients requiring parenteral nutrition. *Gastroenterology*, **80**, 103–7.

Maki, D. G., Weiss, C. F. and Sarafin, H. W. (1977) A semi-quantitative culture method for identifying intravenous catheter related infection. *New England Journal of Medicine*, **296**, 1305–9.

Messing, B., Beiiah, M., Giarard-Papau, F., Leleve, D. and Bernier, J. J. (1982) Technical hazards of using nutritive mixtures in bags for cyclical parenteral nutrition in 48 gastroenterological patients. *Gut*, **23**, 297–303.

Mughall, M. and Irving, M. (1986) Home parenteral nutrition in the United Kingdom. *Lancet*, **ii**, 383–7.

Peters, C. and Fischer, J. E. (1980) Studies on calorie to nitrogen ratio for total parenteral nutrition. *Surgery, Gynaecology and Obstetrics*, **151**, 1–8.

Peters, J. L., Belshan, B. A., Taylor, B. A and Watt-Smith, S. (1984) Long-term venous access. *British Journal of Hospital Medicine*, **32**, 230–42.

Pettigrew, R. A., Lang, S. D. R., Haydock, B. A., Parry, B. R., Bremner, D. A. and Hill, G. L. (1985) Catheter related sepsis in patients on intravenous nutrition: a prospective study of quantitative catheter cultures and guidewire changes for suspected sepsis. *British Journal of Surgery*, **72**, 52–5.

Phillips, G. B. and Odgers, C. L. (1982) Parenteral nutrition, current status and concepts. *Drugs*, **23**, 276–323.

Robinovitvh, A. E. (1981) Home total parenteral nutrition: a psychosocial viewpoint. *Journal of Parenteral and Enteral Nutrition*, **5**, 522–5.

Roslyn, J. H., Pitt, H. A., Mann, L. L., Ament, M. E. and Bestan, L. (1983) Gall bladder disease in patients on long-term parenteral nutrition. *Gastroenterology*, **84**, 148–54.

164 References

Shike, M., Harrison, J. E., Sturtridge, W. C., Tam, C. S., Bobechko, P. E., Jones, G., Murray, T. M. and Jeejeebhoy, K. N. (1980) Metabolic bone disease in patients receiving long-term total parenteral nutrition. *Annals of Internal Medicine*, **92**, 343–50.

Shmitz, J. E., Dolp, R., Grunert, A. and Ahnefeld, F. W. (1982) The effects of solutions of varying branch chain concentrations on the plasma amino acid pattern and metabolism in intensive care patients. *Clinical Nutrition*, **1**, 147–58.

Williamson, R. C. N. (1984) Disuse atrophy of the intestinal tract. *Clinical Nutrition*, **3**, 169–70.

Wood, S. R., Kendall, G. P. N. and Rodrigues, C. A. (1985) Placement of a tunnelled catheter with a fixed hub using a split introducer. *British Journal of Parenteral Therapy*, **6**, 96–9.

Woods, H. F. and Alberti, K. J. N. M. (1972) Dangers of intravenous fructose. *Lancet*, **ii**, 1354–7.

7

NUTRITION
IN DISEASE

7.1 Gastrointestinal disease

7.1.1 THE OESOPHAGUS

Two common oesophageal disorders have important nutritional implications.

(a) Peptic oesophagitis

This follows gastro-oesophageal reflux due to a defective oesophageal sphincter. The oesophageal mucosa is damaged by gastric secretions and bile acids. The inflamed mucosa may lead to blood loss and ultimately to a fibrotic stricture.

(b) Oesophageal carcinoma

Carcinoma arising in the oesophageal mucosa will also narrow the lumen and bleed.

Both diseases frequently cause dysphagia initially for solid foods and are thereafter accompanied by anaemia. Dysphagia tends to progress more rapidly in patients with oesophageal carcinoma who are more likely to be anorectic and malnourished.

Traditionally patients with dysphagia are given a soft or liquid diet. The latter may consist of a conventional pulverized hospital diet which is visually unattractive. When a patient is unable to swallow ordinary food the restoration and maintenance of nutritional status, pending treatment of the cause of dysphagia, may best be achieved by the use of the polymeric liquid diets discussed in Chapter 5. Limitation of nutrient intake by anorexia or altered taste sensation can often be overcome by the passage of a fine bore naso-gastric feeding tube through the stenosis for naso-gastric feeding by continuous infusion thereby relieving the patient of the responsibility of eating. Under these circumstances an X-ray is essential to confirm the enterogastric position of the catheter before feeding is commenced. Parenteral nutrition which is more expensive and hazardous is less commonly needed in these patients.

7.1.2 GASTRIC AND DUODENAL DISEASE

(a) Peptic ulcer disease

Iron deficiency is quite common due to chronic blood loss, and additional iron supplements may be needed. Occasionally malnutrition accompanies the anorexia which occurs in gastric ulcer disease or vomiting caused by ulcers in the region of the pylorus. The latter leads to fluid and electrolyte imbalance which is more important than any nutritional deficit. Nutritional status is usually restored after definitive treatment of the ulcer, but very rarely parenteral nutrition may be required to facilitate the surgical treatment of malnourished patients with pyloric stenosis. Contrary to historical teaching and popular belief there is no role for ulcer diets: these are without benefit in terms of ulcer healing or symptom relief.

(b) Atrophic gastritis

Atrophic gastritis is a form of auto-immune disease which is characterized by mucosal atrophy and lymphocytic infiltration. Some patients have associated disorders such as vitiligo, thyroid disease, and adrenal insufficiency. There is a higher incidence of gastric cancer in patients with this condition. From a nutritional standpoint there are three implications:

● The loss of secretion of intrinsic factor leads to malabsorption of Vitamin B12. Because of large hepatic stores patients do not present with pernicious anaemia for many years. Intramuscular replacement of this vitamin is then required

● Loss of acid secretion facilitates bacterial colonization of the small intestine and thus malabsorption. This is a recognized cause of malnutrition in elderly subjects

● Some patients develop iron deficiency. Impaired absorption and increased iron loss may be implicated when iron supplements are needed

(c) Gastric cancer

Gastric cancer has a poor prognosis as patients may have few symptoms until their disease is advanced. Some patients present with anaemia and weight loss, malnutrition or cachexia. Under these circumstances pre-operative nutritional support is required and will have to be continued in the post-operative period.

Naso-gastric feeding can be used pre-operatively except in patients with gastric outlet obstruction who need parenteral feeding. Parenteral nutrition will frequently be required in the post-operative period, particularly in the malnourished patient, to prevent further protein wasting until the enteral route is available.

(d) Gastric surgery

There is a spectrum of surgical intervention, and the choice of operation is governed by the nature of the disease. This includes highly selective vagotomy, vagotomy and drainage, vagotomy and antrectomy, polyagastrectomy, and complete gastrectomy. These operations cause a variable reduction in acid and intrinsic factor secretion, loss of capacitance, and the loss of the pyloric break depending upon the magnitude of surgery. They have important nutritional implications although minimal disturbance follows highly selective vagotomy and significant problems following conventional vagotomy and drainage are unusual.

(i) Dumping syndrome The dumping syndrome is an unfortunate sequel to partial gastrectomy in some patients. Early dumping is due to hypovolaemia associated with the rapid emptying of the hypertonic nutrient solution into the small intestine. The rapid absorption of carbohydrate stimulates excessive insulin secretion and this may

subsequently lead to hypoglycaemia which characterizes the late dumping syndrome.

Both of these problems can be reduced by instructing the patient to eat small frequent meals, to avoid highly refined carbohydrates, and not to take fluids with or shortly after food.

(ii) Reduced food intake A reduced appetite, early satiety, and intolerance of large meals are other features of gastric resection. Reduced food intake can cause malnutrition as the effect of dietary restriction is compounded by mild malabsorption. The importance of frequent meals should be emphasized. Supplements of iron, Vitamin B12, and in some patients Vitamin D, may have to be given.

7.1.3 DISEASES OF THE SMALL INTESTINE

Disease of the small intestine leads to malabsorption. The physiology of digestion and absorption is discussed in Chapter 2 and the causes of malabsorption are reviewed in Chapter 4, so this section is confined to the nutritional management of small bowel disease. First it is worth considering two general points relating to malabsorption, or more specifically steatorrhoea. Unabsorbed fatty acids form complexes with calcium which free oxalate and this is subsequently absorbed through the colon. Patients with steatorrhoea and intact colons are thus prone to form oxalate renal calculi. This tendency can be reduced by the avoidance of oxalate-rich foods such as rhubarb and strawberries and the administration of supplements of 2–3 g of calcium. Dietary fat reduction is also of value. Secondly the limitation of dietary fat, with or without medium chain triglyceride substitution, can substantially improve symptoms by reducing diarrhoea. However it is then necessary to increase the carbohydrate energy supply.

(a) Gluten enteropathy

Some patients develop an immunological response to gluten which damages the small intestinal mucosa resulting in partial or sub-total villous atrophy. The degradation of gluten in the intestinal lumen means that the proximal small intestine is maximally affected. The disease may present in childhood when solid food is added to the diet, or during the course of adult life. Recognition may follow the development of anaemia due to iron or folate deficiency caused by proximal small bowel damage. Alternatively the patient may present with the features of malabsorption. This is a consequence of extensive mucosal disease and the loss of mucosal synthesis of cholecystokinin, and thus impaired biliary and pancreatic secretion.

There are two aspects of the nutritional management of gluten enteropathy. Firstly the patient must adhere to a strict gluten-free diet which will allow the intestinal mucosa to recover. Secondly specific nutrient deficiency and protein energy malnutrition may require correction.

(i) Gluten-free diet As discussed in Chapter 3, 7–15% of wheat flour consists of protein, 90% of which is gluten. The relationship of other cereals to wheat is shown in Fig. 7.1. Rye and barley should also be excluded. Oats are less likely to cause problems but they may need to be avoided by some patients. Rice and maize are harmless.

The exclusion of gluten leads to a rapid recovery of symptoms and mucosal damage in children. Recovery takes longer in adults in whom less severe mucosal damage may persist. The reintroduction of gluten, deliberate or unintentional, leads to a rapid symptomatic relapse.

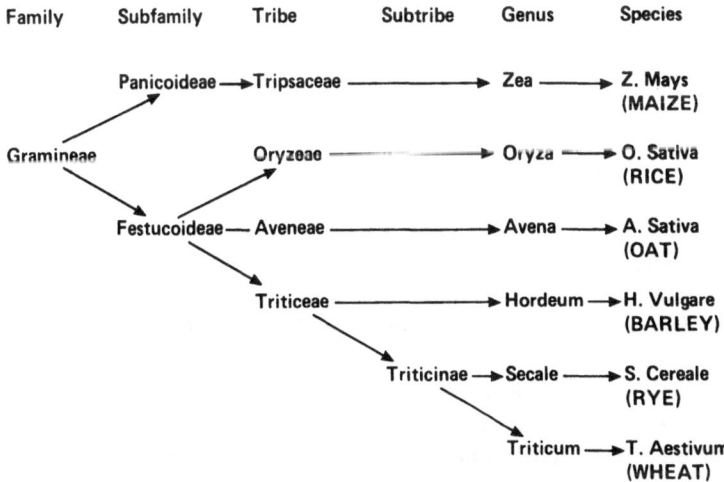

Figure 7.1 The relationship of wheat to other cereals. Adapted from Kasarda *et. al.* (1978), *Perspectives in coeliac disease*, MTP Press, Lancaster

(ii) Correction of nutrient deficiencies The brunt of the damage occurs in the proximal small bowel so iron and folate supplements may be needed. Malabsorption of fat soluble vitamins may occur in patients with steatorrhoea, and some develop muscular cramps due to hypocalcaemia associated with Vitamin D deficiency. Prior to small bowel biopsy it is also prudent to measure the prothrombin time as an index of Vitamin K status. Specific nutrient replacement therapy is no longer required when mucosal recovery has occurred.

Significant protein energy malnutrition is uncommon in gluten enteropathy. It occurs when patients fail to comply with a gluten-free diet, with severe disease, and in the presence of complications such as ulcerative jejuno-ileitis. The use of enteral supplements with gluten and lactose-free polymeric diets is helpful in some of these patients. Peptide diets with medium chain triglycerides such as Peptisorbon are theoretically attractive for reasons which are discussed in Chapter 5. Other patients may need parenteral nutrition pending mucosal recovery under the influence of other treatment such as corticosteroid therapy.

(b) Crohn's disease

Crohn's disease is a segmental full thickness inflammatory disease which may occur anywhere in the intestinal tract, but its effects are usually more severe in the small intestine. The nutritional impact of Crohn's disease may be substantial, and it is a common cause of protein energy malnutrition. Patients frequently reduce their food intake because of anorexia or in an attempt to reduce symptoms such as abdominal pain and diarrhoea. The food that is eaten may be malabsorbed because of extensive disease, bacterial over-growth complicating stricture formation, the loss of bile acids due to ileal disease, and the loss of the ileal break through removal of the ileocaecal valve. At the same time nutrient requirements may be enhanced by extensive inflammatory disease and associated sepsis.

There are two aspects of the nutritional management of Crohn's disease: the restoration of nutritional status and the manipulation of the diet to facilitate reduced disease activity. The latter is a source of controversy.

(i) Nutritional support Good dietetic advice may circumvent anorexia and the reduction of dietary fat with or without supplements of

medium chain triglycerides can reduce the symptoms of steatorrhoea. Nevertheless some patients with severe disease need supplemental naso-gastric feeding with either polymeric or chemically defined diets. Polymeric diets are cheaper, elemental diets are favoured by some clinicians, peptide diets may be more readily absorbed. Much work is needed to define the relative merits of the different types of liquid feeds in this context, and the subject is discussed more fully in Chapter 5. Whichever nutrient is selected long-term supplemental naso-gastric feeding by home nocturnal naso-gastric hyperalimentation helps many patients with borderline intestinal function.

Crohn's disease is an important indication for parenteral nutrition. This is frequently needed in the short term to restore nutritional status or to tide the patient over a period of intestinal failure or surgery. Long-term treatment is necessary in patients who have severe and extensive disease, particularly in those with residual short bowel following resection. Crohn's disease is the commonest indication for home parenteral nutrition in the United Kingdom, and this subject is discussed in Chapter 6.

(ii) Diet and disease activity The cause of Crohn's disease is unknown. The suggestion that it represents a reaction to dietary components, allergic or otherwise, has attracted interest. It seems unlikely that food components instigate the inflammatory response but they may increase the inflammation in diseased bowel. This concept led to the introduction of bowel rest therapy initially by total parenteral nutrition. Undoubtedly some patients resistant to other forms of treatment go into remission when food is withdrawn. The relative importance of dietary exclusion or more effective nutritional support by the parenteral route remains to be established. More recently the concept of bowel rest has been extended by the exclusive use of elemental and thus hypoallergenic diets such as Vivonex. In some series this preparation has been found equivalent to conventional steroid therapy for suppressing disease activity. In the author's experience the bouquet, flavour and after-taste of this product are so offensive that it can only be reliably administered by naso-gastric tube. Nevertheless it is a useful alternative to parenteral nutrition.

When these measures have led to a reduction of disease activity some authorities then employ an exclusion diet. This is a basic and very limited diet which is described in Chapter 8 and illustrated in

Table 8.3. Food items which have been most commonly associated with recurrent symptoms are excluded. These include wheat, dairy produce, coffee and food additives. Once established on the exclusion diet the patient reintroduces different items individually in a predetermined order every three days and in this way identifies any food intolerance. This diet is quite unsuitable for patients who are malnourished or who have severe disease. Furthermore it cannot be assessed in patients who are asymptomatic.

(c) Miscellaneous small intestinal disorders

Radiation enteritis which usually follows treatment for pelvic malignancy, bacterial over-growth which is discussed in Chapter 4, and tropical sprue all impair intestinal function, lead to malabsorption and ultimately malnutrition.

Patients with radiation enteritis are difficult to treat. Nutritional supplements may be helpful but some require parenteral nutrition, often for prolonged periods. Folate supplements are needed in addition to antibiotics for patients with tropical sprue.

(d) Intestinal resection and the short bowel syndrome

Patients may undergo massive intestinal resection on account of Crohn's disease, volvulus, or mesenteric vascular occlusion which may be arterial or venous. Physiological factors relating to the short bowel and intestinal adaption are considered in Chapter 2. Three principles govern the nutritional management of the patient with short bowel syndrome. These are the maintenance of nutrition, the relief of symptoms, and the encouragement of intestinal adaption.

Patients should receive enteral feeding otherwise adaption will not take place. Whereas total parenteral nutrition may lead to mucosal atrophy, in the presence of malnutrition supplemental parenteral nutrition facilitates adaption. Many patients find small frequent meals of conventional food preferable to liquid diets, and if liquid diets are employed they should be given in addition to conventional meals. The relative merits of polymeric, peptic and elemental diets remains to be established by clinical trial. Traditionally, low lactose and very low fat diets with medium chain triglycerides are prescribed. In many patients lactose restriction may be unnecessary, and studies which have investigated the role of fat have failed to demonstrate symptomatic improvement with severe fat restriction. Furthermore evidence is accumulating that long-chain fatty acids promote intestinal adaption.

Patients in whom the residual intestine is too short or diseased will need to continue on supplemental parenteral nutrition and should be considered for home parenteral nutrition. Adaption will continue in some of these and ultimately they may be able to dispense with intravenous feeding after many months.

In the initial stages of treatment deficiencies of calcium, magnesium, zine, and iron frequently require correction, and vitamin replacement is needed. H_2 antagonists help to block the enhanced gastric secretion which impairs digestion, and pancreatic supplements and Codeine Phosphate are helpful.

(e) Enterocutaneous fistulae

Formerly enterocutaneous fistulae involving the small intestine were associated with high mortality. The development of parenteral nutrition has transformed the outlook for these patients who no longer die of intestinal failure. The use of total parenteral nutrition with bowel rest therapy allows many fistulae to close, and depending on the site of the fistula, elemental and peptide diets may also be effective. Even if the fistula fails to close the patient can be satisfactorily maintained until surgery is planned. This is necessary for subjects with distal stenosis and for most with active Crohn's disease.

(f) Jejuno-ileal bypass surgery

The anastomosis of 30 cm of proximal jejunum to 10 cm of distal ileum is a very effective remedy for morbid obesity. It leads to anorexia and malabsorption which ensures weight loss. Unfortunately the development of cirrhosis is an unacceptably common sequel to this operation and many patients have died of liver failure. This form of surgical intervention has fallen into disrepute.

7.1.4 DISEASES OF THE LARGE INTESTINE

(a) Ulcerative colitis

There is no convincing evidence that diet has any role in the development of this disease at least in adults. In contrast to Crohn's disease bowel rest therapy is not effective in the management of acute disease. The apparent improvement which occasionally accompanies milk withdrawal may reflect temporary hypolactasia.

Malnutrition is relatively uncommon although some patients may require peri-operative nutritional support. There is some evidence that Sulphasalazine which is principally used for maintenance treatment impairs folate absorption. Supplements may be required in patients who have poor diets.

(b) Irritable bowel syndrome

This is a very common but poorly defined condition which involves abnormal motility of both large and small intestine. It is characterized by abnormal bowel habit, constipation or constipation alternating with diarrhoea, abdominal pain and abdominal distension.

Nutritional management involves the use of high fibre diets, and the exploration of possible food intolerance. The latter is a source of controversy.

High fibre diets relieve constipation in most but not all sufferers, but they do not help the other symptoms. In some patients these appear to be provoked or aggravated by specific food items. The exploration of possible food intolerance is discussed in the next chapter. However it is important to remember that this diagnostic label is frequently applied to patients whose symptoms are psychosomatic. The potential abuse of limited diets in this population is obvious.

(c) Diverticular disease

Diverticular disease is a condition in which the mucosal lining herniates through weak points in the colonic wall to form pouches. The bowel wall becomes shorter and thicker and the colonic lumen narrower. Increased intraluminal pressures have been demonstrated and inflammation may occur in the diverticulae.

The disease is uncommon in underdeveloped societies where the diet is rich in fibre. It is common in the Western world where a lov fibre diet is consumed. Within Western societies it becomes more prevalent with age and is less common in vegetarians. Dietary surveys suggest that people with the disease eat less fibre, especially cereal fibre, than control subjects. Fibre-depleted diets in animals produce changes in colonic pressures which are similar to those found in patients. Consequently diverticular disease is regarded as a fibre deficiency syndrome.

Whereas in the early part of this century physicians were recommending high fibre diets for the management of this disease the opposing view was subsequently advocated and widely upheld. Painter and Birkitt stimulated the current interest in fibre in 1971 and now high fibre diets are regarded as standard treatment.

Fibre intake should be increased from the average 20 g to 40 g a day slowly over a 4-week period. Maximum therapeutic benefit is not obtained for three months. Symptomatic improvement is matched by reduced colonic pressures, and there is some evidence to suggest that complications such as diverticulitis and perforation are reduced.

(d) Colonic cancer

Colon cancer like diverticular disease occurs more commonly in subjects who eat a Western-style diet. There is an inverse relationship between the ingestion of vegetables and particularly the pentose fraction of dietary fibre and the risk of colon cancer. The ingestion of fibre increases faecal bulk and this appears to relate to the intake of pentose from different cereal sources. This leads to the suggestion that high fibre diets protect against cancer by diluting or binding faecal carcinogens. It is also likely that such diets reduce intestinal transit time and modify the luminal microflora. No significant relationship has been found between bowel cancer and the consumption of meat and fat which enhance biliary bile acid secretion.

Clearly nutrition plays no part in the management of this disease, but patients who undergo surgery and develop complications may require temporary parenteral feeding.

7.2 Diseases of the pancreas

7.2.1 ACUTE PANCREATITIS

Acute pancreatitis is a dangerous disease which may result from gall stone impaction or follow an alcoholic binge. Autodigestion by activated pancreatic enzymes can lead to haemorrhagic pancreatitis with necrosis and peritonitis. Thus it is important to avoid pancreatic stimulation by naso-gastric aspiration, and H_2 blockade is helpful in reducing gastric secretion. Clearly oral or enteral feeding is contra-indicated and parenteral nutrition should be instituted early especially in those patients who are already malnourished. Peripheral parenteral nutrition may suffice for well-nourished patients with moderate disease.

7.2.2 CHRONIC PANCREATITIS

Chronic pancreatitis leads to exocrine insufficiency and thus malabsorption. Many patients suffer pain and are reluctant to eat. Consequently chronic pancreatitis is associated with malnutrition.

The prescription of pancreatic supplements is routine and these are rendered more effective by H_2 antagonists. Patients should abstain from alcohol. For reasons which have been discussed in Section 7.1.3 dietary restriction of fat may improve symptoms and reduce oxaluria. Medium chain triglycerides are sometimes well tolerated, and the addition of carbohydrate and protein supplements (which are discussed in Chapter 5) helps patients who are malnourished. Additional fat soluble vitamins may have to be given.

Naso-gastric feeding allows additional nutritional support particularly for the anorectic patient, and liquid diets in which the majority of fat is supplied as medium chain triglycerides e.g. Trisorbon may be preferable. Some patients need parenteral feeding. The suggestion that total parenteral nutrition with prolonged bowel rest improves the course of this disease requires further study.

7.2.3 MISCELLANEOUS DISORDERS OF THE PANCREAS

Cystic fibrosis is a multi-system disease and a common cause of pancreatic exocrine insufficiency. It is discussed later in this chapter. Diabetes mellitus is considered in the next section.

7.3 Diabetes mellitus

7.3.1 THE SPECTRUM OF DIABETES

Diabetes is a complex metabolic disease which is arbitrarily defined on the basis of elevated blood glucose concentration. Patients with values equal to or greater than 7 mmol per litre in fasting venous blood or

10 mmol per litre after a glucose challenge are defined as diabetics. Two types of diabetes are recognized, idiopathic insulin-dependent diabetes and maturity onset diabetes.

In idiopathic insulin-dependent diabetes there are inherited factors which are HLA linked and related to the immune response system; environmental factors probably include viral infections. These patients suffer a failure of pancreatic insulin secretion which may represent an auto-immune disorder of the islet cells. Non-insulin-dependent diabetes otherwise known as maturity onset diabetes is unrelated to the HLA system or viral infections but there is a strong inherited tendency. Insulin levels are normal or increased, there is an impaired response to glucose and increased insulin resistance. This form of diabetes frequently co-exists with obesity which may act as a diabetogenic environmental factor in those who are genetically predisposed. Obesity has important implications for dietary management.

Hyperglycaemia is the feature which leads to the diagnosis of diabetes and which may be directly responsible for an osmotic diuresis and dehydration. Nevertheless it is only one of a spectrum of abnormalities. The loss of insulin leads to reduced uptake in oxidation of glucose in muscle, reduced muscle glycogen, and release of amino acids including alanine which is transported to the liver for gluconeogenesis. There is reduced fatty acid uptake in adipose tissue and increased lipolysis. Reduced glucose uptake by adipose tissue leads to a reduction of glycerophosphate in triglycerides for fatty acid synthesis. Many of these abnormalities which persists after treatment are shown in Table 7.1. These collectively lead to the problems of vascular disease, renal disease, retinopathy and neuropathy which characterize diabetic morbidity.

7.3.2 DIETARY MANAGEMENT

Careful dietary management is crucial for diabetic patients. Some are controlled by diet alone, others by diet and insulin or diet and drugs. Traditionally diabetes was regarded as a disorder of carbohydrate tolerance. For a long time it was treated by carbohydrate restriction with little attention being paid to the nature of the glycaemic response to different types of carbohydrate food. Furthermore carbohydrate restriction led to increased fat consumption which may have enhanced the development of vascular disease in these patients.

Table 7.1 Abnormalities in controlled diabetes*

Plasma
  Carbohydrate
    Glucose ↑
  Lipids
    FFA ketones ↑
    Tg VLDL ↑
    Cholesterol LDL ↑
    HDL ↓
  Proteins
    Branch chain amino acids ↑
    Alanine ↑
    Glycosylated proteins ↑
    Viscosity ↑
    Fibrinolysis ↓
Cells
  Erythrocytes
    Glycosylated Hb ↑
    O₂ Affinity ↑
    Deformability ↓
  Leukocytes
    Chemotaxis ↓
    Phagocytosis ↓
  Platelets
    Aggregation ↑
    Adhesiveness ↑

*(Adapted from Baird, J. D. Diet and Diabetes Mellitus. In: *Nutrition and Health*, M. R. Turner (ed.) M.T.P. Press, ch. 10, 135–47)

(a) Carbohydrate

After controlling the hyperglycaemia most diabetologists now supply 60% of the dietary energy as carbohydrate. This should be in the form of complex carbohydrate with fibre, so that glucose and sucrose are avoided. This is effectively a slow release preparation which avoids sudden post-prandial glucose peaks. In this respect viscous fibre sources such as pectin and guar are more effective than fibrous fibre such as bran. Thus improved diabetic control may be achieved with foods such as legumes and fruits which are rich in these substances or by using guar gum obtained from the Indian cluster bean as a pharmacological additive. Unfortunately many patients resent the viscous sensation of this material.

(b) Fat

Contrary to previous practice only 20–25% of the total energy is provided in this form, and 30–50% of this fat should be polyunsaturated.

(c) Total energy

Many patients with non-insulin-dependent diabetes are obese. Obesity increases insulin resistance and weight loss improves diabetic control. It therefore follows that energy-restricted diets are required for many patients. Weight loss appears difficult in these patients and can only be achieved by careful counselling. High fibre diets are helpful by increasing satiety.

The energy intake will need to be adjusted in the insulin-dependent diabetic according to the anticipated physical activity. Additional carbohydrate is needed before embarking on unaccustomed exercise.

(d) Dietary composition

If a patient requires 2000 kcal (8.4 MJ), 60% of this energy should be given as unrefined carbohydrate. The patient will therefore receive 1200 kcal (5.04 MJ) in this form which is equivalent to 300 g of carbohydrate. This can be selected from food lists of 10 g carbohydrate exchanges. The same patient may need 15% of the total energy as protein. Thus 300 kcal (1.2 MJ) are supplied in this form, equivalent to 75 g of protein. Similarly 55 g of fat are needed to supply 25% of the energy needs or 500 kcal (2.1 MJ) and at least one third of this should be polyunsaturated.

(e) Daily distribution of the diet

The distribution of the diet throughout the day will depend on the nature of the diabetes and the lifestyle and needs of the individual patient. In normal practice three patterns emerge, which are summarized in Table 7.2.

- The labile insulin dependent diabetic who receives more than one injection of insulin a day will require three main meals and three snacks
- The stable insulin dependent diabetic who receives a single daily insulin injection may only need a bedtime snack in addition to the three main meals
- The stable non-insulin dependent diabetic who frequently needs to lose weight should only require the three main meals

Table 7.2   The distribution of the diet in different types of diabetes

Patient group	Distribution of the diet					
	Breakfast	Snack	Lunch	Snack	Dinner	Snack
Labile insulin dependent	$\frac{1}{10}$	$\frac{1}{10}$	$\frac{2}{10}$	$\frac{1}{10}$	$\frac{3}{10}$	$\frac{1}{10}$
Stable insulin dependent	$\frac{2}{7}$		$\frac{2}{7}$		$\frac{2}{7}$	$\frac{1}{7}$
*Stable non-insulin dependent	$\frac{2}{7}$		$\frac{2}{7}$		$\frac{3}{7}$	

*Evening snack may be required by some patients receiving sulphonyurea drugs

7.4 Diseases of the liver

The liver has important metabolic functions. These include blood glucose homeostasis, bile secretion, protein synthesis and detoxification. They are variably disturbed in diseases which affect the liver. Patients with severe disease are at risk of hypoglycaemia, haemorrhagic diathesis and encephalopathy. Acute liver disease is commonly due to drugs and viral hepatitis. There are more significant nutritional implications for patients with chronic liver disease. Metastatic and alcoholic liver disease are frequently associated with malnutrition. The subjects of alcohol abuse and cancer are discussed in later sections.

7.4.1 ACUTE LIVER DISEASE

There are no specific nutritional implications for patients with acute viral hepatitis. The historical advice to avoid fatty food has no scientific foundation, indeed in one study patients fared better when the diet contained fat. Care must be taken to ensure a sufficient supply of carbohydrate particularly during the period of anorexia. Patients with fulminant liver failure will require intravenous dextrose to prevent hypoglycacmia as well as other forms of intensive management which are beyond the scope of this book.

7.4.2 CHRONIC LIVER DISEASE

(a) Carbohydrate

Patients with severe chronic liver disease and hepatic decompensation need an adequate supply of energy from carbohydrate (40 kcal/kg) preferably delivered in six feeds a day. This reduces the risk of hypoglycaemia and the production of ammonia by suppressing the deamination of amino acids from food and muscle protein.

Adequate carbohydrate consumption must also be ensured in patients with hepatic porphyrias. During attacks high carbohydrate diets suppress ALA synthase and reduce porphyrin synthesis.

(b) Protein

Protein should be restricted in encephalopathic patients who should receive 0.3 to 0.8 g/kg i.e. 20 to 60 g according to tolerance. It is withdrawn from patients in coma. Traditionally protein of high biological value is used to supply essential amino acids to reduce the total protein needs and ammonia formation. However some amino acids have a greater ammonigenic potential because they are deaminated and not transaminated in body tissue. These include glycine, threanine, glutamine, lycine, and asparagine. They are found in greater concentration in egg and meat than in milk. Some workers have demonstrated better protein tolerance using vegetable proteins. More work is required to assess the relative merits of different protein sources as well as a potential role of additional essential amino acids or their alpha keto analogues.

Protein tolerance can be improved by the administration of Lactulose. This appears to act as an energy substrate for intestinal micro-organisms which subsequently utilize nitrogenous waste products. The use of this preparation allows the patient to take more protein in the diet which facilitates nutritional management.

Much interest has focussed on the abnormal plasma amino acid profiles which are found in cirrhotic subjects. Typically there is a reduction of branch chain amino acids, possibly due to hyper-insulinaemia. Because of shared transport mechanisms it is postulated that this encourages uptake by the central nervous system of increased amounts of other amino acids which may lead to the formation of false neurotransmitters. Based on this theory branch chain enriched amino acid solutions have been prepared for enteral and parenteral nutrition. The former are discussed in Chapter 5. These solutions may allow a positive nitrogen balance to be achieved with no deterioration in mental function but further work is needed to clarify this potential clinical role.

(c) Lipid

Concern about the use of Intralipid in patients with chronic liver disease who are prone to portal systemic encephalopathy would appear to be unjustified. The reduced lipid clearance in such patients is not significant, neither is the effect of increased free tryptophan following displacement from albumin by fatty acids produced by the peripheral metabolism of lipid. Conversely it may be argued that a reduction in circulating insulin following the substitution of some dextrose for lipid might be expected to improve plasma amino acid profiles, particularly branch chain amino acid concentrations.

(d) Vitamins

Patients with prolonged cholestasis will need supplements of fat soluble Vitamins A, K, and D, and this particularly applies to those with primary biliary cirrhosis. Alcoholic subjects may need additional B vitamins which should be given before commencing dextrose infusion.

(e) Electrolytes

Sodium restriction is required in ascitic or oedematous patients. A diet containing 50 mmol of sodium is reasonably palatable. Caution should be exercised with salt substitutes which contain potassium. Many cirrhotic patients receive Spironolactone or other potassium-conserving diuretics and their ability to excrete potassium may be further impaired by the hepato-renal syndrome.

7.5 Alcohol-related disease

7.5.1 ALCOHOL CONSUMPTION

The adjusted price of alcoholic beverages in Britain has been reduced by half since the end of the Second World War and the per capita annual consumption has increased to approximately 10 litres a year. Whereas present consumption is marginally less than at the beginning of this century and substantially less than estimates of alcohol intake at the beginning of the previous century, consumption is now increasing significantly especially among women. An increase in the incidence of alcohol-related disease such as cirrhosis has followed. These problems occur more frequently in the EEC countries where alcohol intake is greater. Alcohol consumption in France is double that reported in Britain.

7.5.2 ALCOHOL AND DISEASE

Excessive alcohol consumption is responsible for a wide range of disease. Liver damage is well known, covering the spectrum of fatty liver, alcoholic hepatitis, and cirrhosis. Acute and chronic pancreatitis may occur. Neurological disease includes peripheral neuropathy, dementia, epilepsy and the thiamin responsive Wernicke-Korsakoff syndrome. Some patients develop cardiomyopathy and others become anaemic. Anaemia may be due to haematinic deficiency, usually folate, but occasionally it is sideroblastic. The foetal alcohol syndrome is a disorder of foetal development characterized by growth deficiency, developmental delay, prematurity, mental retardation, microcephaly, and various facial, limb and cardiac defects. These have been attributed to the *in utero* effects of heavy maternal ethanol consumption of 90 g a day, however moderate drinking has not been shown to be harmless. Many of the problems of alcohol abuse relate to trauma and psychological effects. After prolonged periods the sudden cessation of heavy consumption leads to delirium tremens characterized by hallucinations, mania, autonomic dysfunction and fits.

7.5.3 ALCOHOL METABOLISM

Ethanol is rapidly absorbed. It is initially metabolized by alcohol dehydrogenase to acetaldehyde. This reaction creates ATP and forms

NaDH which is reoxidized by a pathway which involves the formation of lactate from pyruvate. In patients who drink regularly microsomal ethanol oxidising enzymes are induced. This pathway also forms acetaldehyde but no ATP. The acetaldehyde is converted to acetyl CoA for entry into the tricarboxylic acid cycle or synthesis of fatty acids or cholesterol.

These metabolic pathways utilize vitamins such as niacin, thiamin and riboflavin. Ethanol metabolism can interrupt carbohydrate and lipid metabolism. Significant hypoglycaemia has long been recognized as a dangerous consequence of excessive ethanol ingestion, especially in the fasted patient. Lactic acidosis is another hazard. However the regular consumpton of a modest ethanol intake equivalent to one to two drinks per day leads to an increase in high-density lipoprotein. This may be advantageous as discussed in Section 7.7.

7.5.4 ALCOHOL AND NUTRITION

Excessive alcohol consumption may have an adverse effect on nutrition through various mechanisms. Nutritional impairment is indirectly aggravated in patients with ethanol-induced liver or pancreatic disease.

(a) Diet

Excessive alcohol consumption induces gastritis which causes anorexia. The diet of many alcoholics is deficient in specific nutrients such as folate. Some alcoholic beverages contain much iron and may lead to siderosis.

(b) Intestinal function

Morphological changes occur in the small intestinal mucosa. There may be impaired absorption of actively transported nutrients and disaccharidase deficiency. Bowel motility is also increased.

Malabsorption of amino acids, folate, thiamin and Vitamin B12 has been documented. More general malabsorption including steatorrhoea follows pancreatic and hepatic damage.

(c) Interaction with nutrients

Alcohol interferes with pyridoxine activation, increases the requirement for some vitamins including thiamin and niacin, and enhances the degradation of activated Vitamin D and hepatic sequestration of folate.

7.6 Cardiovascular disease

In Western societies the relationship of nutrition to cardiovascular disease is usually one of over-provision with particular reference to saturated fats and sodium. Elsewhere deficiency syndromes are more important. Thiamin deficiency is responsible for wet beri-beri in some underdeveloped countries, and selenium deficiency causes a cardiomyopathy in parts of China. Selenium deficiency has also been reported in patients who have been treated by prolonged total parenteral nutrition without supplements. These disorders are discussed in more detail in Chapter 4.

7.6.1 ISCHAEMIC HEART DISEASE

Ischaemic heart disease gained prominence in the USA and Europe in the 1920s, and there has been a massive increase in the incidence since the Second World War. Whereas the incidence in the USA has fallen 20% from a very high level in the 1960s, rates in the United Kingdom remain near the top of the world league table, while increases are being observed in Eastern Europe, Sweden and Russia. This is the dominant cause of death in males from the 30 year age group upwards and it kills 9% by the age of 65. Rates are much lower in women in whom the disease is not common before the age of 60 years.

(a) Factors associated with the development of ischaemic heart disease

Factors associated with the development of ischaemic heart disease, many of which are interrelated, are shown in Table 7.3. The three big risk factors appear to be hypertension, cigarette smoking, and serum concentration of low density lipoprotein (or total) cholesterol. Professional men now have a below average risk of death from this disease

Table 7.3 Factors associated with the development of ischaemic heart disease

---

Age
Sex
Social class
Cigarette smoking
Blood pressure
Blood lipids
Physical activity
Obesity
Glucose intolerance
Family history
Personality type
Blood-clotting factors
Diet

---

in contrast to unskilled labourers. Physical activity is important in some studies, the effect of obesity may be mediated through blood pressure, diabetes, and blood lipids, and the influence of family history is in part through the major risk factors. Some studies suggest that the striving obsessional 'type A' personality is particularly susceptible. Recently more attention is being paid to the influence of blood clotting mechanisms.

(b) Diet and ischaemic heart disease

(i) Cholesterol An international study of 18 populations in seven countries over 10 years involving 12 000 men showed a clear association between diet, serum cholesterol, and the incidence of ischaemic heart disease. Cholesterol is a component of atheromatous plaque, high serum cholesterol concentrations are associated with the development of atheroma in individual patients, and serum cholesterol values correlate with the consumption of saturated fat.

The increase in serum cholesterol that follows the consumption of saturated fats is mainly due to palmitic and to a lesser extent stearic acids. Medium chain triglycerides, although they are saturated, and monounsaturated fats do not influence serum cholesterol values. Polyunsaturated fats lower the serum cholesterol. However a reduction in serum cholesterol can be achieved more readily by reducing saturated fat consumption than by substituting poly-unsaturated fats, although both changes may be desirable for practical dietetic reasons. Dietary cholesterol has little influence on serum values but it is usually consumed in foods which are rich in saturated fat.

Other dietary factors which influence cholesterol are of uncertain significance. Calcium, vanadium, copper, and Vitamin C all depress serum values, which are increased by an excess of Vitamin D.

(ii) Thrombotic tendency Recent interest has focussed on another aspect of the role of diet in ischaemic heart disease. There is evidence to suggest that the thrombotic tendency is increased by long chain fatty acids and reduced by linoleic and arachidonic acid. Patients with ischaemic heart disease have higher plasma values of some clotting factors, notably factor 7, whereas lower values are found in vegetarians who have a lower incidence of this disease. These values can be reduced by feeding high fibre diets.

Dietary factors may also influence platelet behaviour. Fish oils lead to changes in the platelet membrane fatty acid composition and reduce the tendency to aggregation.

(iii) Dietary surveys Surveys have indicated certain dietary factors which may be associated with decreased coronary risk. These include a high total food energy intake, high cereal fibre intake, moderate alcohol consumption, the regular consumption of fish and a high ratio of polyunsaturated to saturated fat. Some forms of fibre such as rolled oats and pectin reduce serum cholesterol values and high fibre diets are accompanied by reduced clotting factor concentrations. Moderate alcohol consumption increases the high density lipoprotein chol-esterol (see Section 7.7) which appears to be protective. The correlation of ischaemic heart disease with a high sucrose con-sumption may reflect the reduced fibre content of such diets or the association of sucrose consumption with saturated fat intake. High dietary sodium may contribute to the development of hypertension in susceptible subjects, and this is discussed in Section 7.6.3. Finally a recent study from the Netherlands demonstrated a 50% reduction in mortality from coronary heart disease in subjects who ate at least 30 g of fish a day.

Table 7.4 Summary of dietary factors associated with ischaemic heart disease

Dietary factor	Influence on risk factor	Incidence of ischaemic heart disease
Sodium	Increased blood pressure	Increased
Saturated fat	Increased sodium cholesterol Increased clotting factors	Increased
Polyunsaturated fats	Reduced serum cholesterol	Reduced
Fibre	Reduced serum cholesterol Reduced clotting factors	Reduced
Moderate alcohol	Increased HDL cholesterol	Reduced
Fish	Uncertain: reduced serum cholesterol and reduced platelet aggregation	Reduced

The influence of the diet on factors related to the development of ischaemic heart disease is summarized in Table 7.4.

7.6.2 CEREBROVASCULAR DISEASE

Risk factors for cerebrovascular disease were assessed in the large Whitehall study of 18 000 male civil servants of 40–64 years. Four risk factors were identified: blood pressure, obesity, cigarette smoking and grade of employment. Systolic blood pressure was found to be a major predictor of stroke, the group in the highest quintile having a fourteenfold greater incidence of stroke. The influence of obesity was not graded according to body mass index, and only men in the highest quintile had a significant and twofold increase in risk. This was due to the influence of hypertension in this group. Hypertension was also the reason for excess risk in lower employment groups. Serum cholesterol was not a risk factor for stroke in contrast to ischaemic heart disease. Other studies have shown that cholesterol is a weaker risk factor for cerebrovascular than ischaemic heart disease.

The role of diet in the development of cerebrovascular disease appears to involve the related problems of hypertension and obesity. Obesity is considered in Section 7.13, and diet in relation to blood pressure is discussed in the following section.

7.6.3 DIET IN HYPERTENSION

(a) Body weight and blood pressure

Many studies have shown an association between obesity and blood pressure. Weight reduction is known to lower blood pressure particularly, but not only, in those patients who are considered to be hypertensive.

(b) Salt and blood pressure

Comparisons between populations have demonstrated a correlation between the level of blood pressure and the amount of salt consumed. Such correlations are less clear in cross-sectional studies within populations. Nevertheless an influence of dietary sodium on blood pressure has been demonstrated in the relatives of hypertensive patients and sodium restriction reduces the blood pressure in hypertensive subjects. This observation was initially made by imposing severe salt restriction as in the Kempner rice/fruit diet which provided 10 mmol of sodium a day. It was unpalatable and therefore impractical. More recent studies have shown that a modest reduction of dietary sodium to 50 mmol is accompanied by a significant reduction in blood pressure and this may be enhanced by feeding a high potassium diet.

The estimated average daily salt intake in Britain is 12 g (200 mmol of sodium) after allowances for salt addition in cooking and at the table. From observed data a reduction of dietary sodium by 50 mmol results in a mean fall in diastolic pressure of 5 mmHg, and further reductions can be obtained by 100 mmol sodium diets or potassium supplementation. Unfortunately such benefits cannot be demonstrated in all patients so this approach remains controversial.

Population surveys in Britain and the USA have shown that 10–15% of middle-aged adults have blood pressure readings in excess of 160/90 mmHg. It has been estimated that a small reduction (2–3 mmHg) in the mean blood pressure would be of major benefit in terms of mortality, currently comparable to that achieved with hypotensive medication. The potential value of sodium restriction is immense. It could save many patients from drug therapy and assist hypertensives who escape detection and possibly patients who develop cardiovascular disease at blood pressures which are currently below the accepted treatment threshold.

7.7 Hyperlipidaemia

7.7.1 THE LIPOPROTEINS

The major lipoproteins are shown in Table 7.5. In the fasting state chylomicrons are absent and 70% of triglyceride is in the form of very low density lipoprotein (VLDL). Most of the plasma cholesterol is in low density lipoprotein fraction 2 (LDL2). High blood lipid values may reflect genetic disorders, the excessive consumption of saturated fats or carbohydrate, and underlying disease.

Table 7.5 The plasma lipoproteins

Class	Subclasses	Major lipids
Chylomicrons		Triglycerides
Very low density lipoproteins (VLDL)		Triglycerides
Low density lipoproteins (LDL)	LDL1	Triglycerides
		Cholesterol ester
	LDL2	Cholesterol ester
High density lipoproteins	HDL2	Phospholipid
		Cholesterol ester
	HDL3	Phospholipid
		Cholesterol ester

7.7.2 LIPOPROTEIN METABOLISM

Chylomicrons are formed during fat absorption by the small intestine. They contain triglycerides with small amounts of cholesterol, phospholipids and apolipoprotein and they enter the circulation via the lymphatic system.

The triglycerides are hydrolyzed by lipoprotein lipase especially in adipose tissue and skeletal muscle. This enzyme is activated by a co-factor which is acquired by the chylomicrons from high density lipoprotein (HDL). Triglyceride hydrolysis results in chylomicrons becoming progressively smaller, surface components such as cholesterol, phospholipid, and co-factor fuse with HDL and the cholesterol rich chylomicron remnant is taken up by the liver.

Very low density lipoproteins (VLDL) are the main transporters of endogenous triglyceride. They are secreted by the liver especially when there is an excessive intake of carbohydrate energy. Hydrolysis by lipoprotein lipase results in smaller LDL1 remnants which are partly removed from the circulation in the splanchnic region and partially converted to LDL2. LDL2 is removed by a receptor mediated process in the peripheral tissues and liver as well as by endocytosis.

LDL is the main transporter of cholesterol. Following receptor uptake cholesterol release suppresses cholesterol synthesis. Cholesterol released in the peripheral tissues is transported back to the liver by HDL following esterification by the enzyme lecithin cholesterol acetyl transferase (LCAT). Patients with familial hypercholesterolaemia suffer an inherited absence of LDL receptors with resulting high LDL2 concentrations.

LDL1 and LDL2 contribute to atherogenesis, HDL protects against atherogenesis, and chylomicrons and VLDL have little effect on arterial disease although chylomicron remnants may be important.

7.7.3 CLINICAL AND NUTRITIONAL ASPECTS OF HYPERLIPIDAEMIA

(a) Hyperchylomicronaemia

Primary hyperchylomicronaemia is due to a deficiency of lipoprotein lipase. This leads to hypertriglyceridaemia. The patient develops eruptive xanthomas, hepatomegaly, and suffers from abdominal pain with or without pancreatitis. Control is achieved by the restriction of dietary fat to 25 g per day, although medium chain triglycerides may be used as they do not depend on chylomicrons for absorption. Alcohol should be avoided.

Secondary hyperchylomicronaemia may complicate diabetic ketoacidosis, alcoholic pancreatitis, or dysgammaglobulinaemia such as occurs in myeloma or systemic lupus erythematosis. Chylomicrons are associated with a turbidity in plasma, but they float to the surface on standing.

(b) Very low density lipoprotein (VLDL)

In the absence of chylomicrons VLDL correlate with serum triglyceride values. Increased VLDL concentration causes a diffuse turbidity, but unlike chylomicrons VLDL does not float to the surface of the plasma or serum on standing.

High VLDL values may be primary and genetically determined or secondary. Secondary hypertriglyceridaemia is associated with high carbohydrate diets, alcohol which may produce very high values in some individuals, obesity, and diseases such as renal failure, diabetes mellitus, hypothyroidism and dysgammaglobulinaemia. As with hyperchylomicronaemia, hypertriglyceridaemia due to high VLDL concentrations is associated with pancreatitis but not with early vascular disease.

Many patients are overweight and triglyceride values can be reduced by weight reduction and restricting the energy supply by carbohydrate to 40% of the total. Alcohol should be avoided.

(c) Low density lipoprotein (LDL)

Patients with familial hypercholesterolaemia lack a functional cell surface lipoprotein receptor which is necessary for the transfer of cholesterol from LDL2. They develop xanthalasmas, premature arcus senilis, and tendon xanthomas. Half of the cases present with early myocardial infarction. Secondary hypercholesterolaemia is a feature of many diverse diseases when it is usually of secondary importance. Examples include prolonged cholestasis such as primary biliary cirrhosis, nephrotic syndrome, chronic renal failure and hypothyroidism.

Dietary management involves a restriction of fat and cholesterol consumption. Patients should eat less than 300 mg of cholesterol a day. Fat should account for less than 30% of the total energy and the ratio of polyunsaturated to saturated fat should be increased from 0.3 to 2.0. This can be achieved by substituting vegetable for animal fat and if necessary soya protein for meat. However, it must be remembered that both palm oil and coconut oil are rich in saturated fats. In addition calorie restriction may be needed in the obese. Plant sterols, for example sitosterol, may lower LDL concentration by reducing cholesterol absorption, and other drugs may be required for example resins like Cholestyramine which bind bile acids and thus enhance cholesterol excretion. These measures lower LDL and thus cholesterol. Further protection may be given by increasing the HDL which can be achieved by moderate alcohol ingestion and regular exercise.

(d) Intermediate density lipoprotein (IDL)

IDL is an intermediate formed in the catabolism of VLDL to LDL which is not usually present in the circulation. It is found in patients with the inborn error of metabolism dysbetaglobulinaemia in whom there is an elevation of serum cholesterol and triglycerides. These people develop palmar and tuberous xanthomas and suffer from severe peripheral vascular disease. Response may be obtained by restricting dietary cholesterol, saturated fats and total calories.

7.8 Renal disease

7.8.1 SPECTRUM OF DISEASE

Many forms of disease both congenital and acquired affect renal function and may lead to renal failure. Acute renal failure is common in hospital practice and can be defined as any condition which results

Table 7.6 Some common causes of renal failure

Acute	Chronic
Pre-renal	Congenital
Gastroenteritis	Polycystic kidneys
Haemorrhage	Medullary cystic kidney disease
Burns	
Sepsis	Primary renal disease
	Glomerulonephritis
Renal	Intestinal nephritis
Shock	Pyelonephritis
Trauma	
Drugs	Obstructive renal disease
Coagulopathies	Ureteric neoplasm
	Bladder neck obstruction
Post-renal	Urethral stricture
Renal stones	
Prostate enlargement	Systemic disease
Renal vascular occlusion	Hypertension
	Diabetes
	Vasculitis
	Analgesic nephropathy

in a sudden fall in the glomerular filtration rate sufficient to cause uraemia. Oliguria with a urine flow of less than 15 ml/min is common, but non-oliguric renal failure may also occur. In chronic renal failure a progressive loss of nephrons leads to a permanent impairment of renal function. Patients move through stages of diminished renal reserve with normal biochemistry, early renal failure when the glomerular filtration rate has fallen to 30 ml per min, to late and end stage renal failure with glomerular filtration rates at 15 and 10 ml/min respectively. The reciprocal plot of the serum creatinine with time has shown that the rate of functional deterioration is linear, and any sudden decline usually denotes an additional problem such as hypovolaemia or drug nephrotoxicity. The common causes of acute and chronic renal failure are shown in Table 7.6.

7.8.2 ACUTE RENAL FAILURE

Management priorities in patients with acute renal failure include restoration of cardiovascular stability, the correction of electrolyte imbalance and the diagnosis and management of the underlying disorder. Following the restoration of cardiovascular and electrolyte status attention should be given to nutritional management.

(a) Energy

The total energy requirements should be met in full to minimize gluconeogenesis with attendant muscle wasting and urea formation. The gastrointestinal tract is unavailable or inadequate in many of these very ill patients who will require total or supplemental parenteral nutrition with dextrose and lipid. Care is required to avoid hypoglycaemia during dialysis in patients who are receiving insulin in dextrose infusions.

(b) Protein

Many physicians supply the estimated nitrogen requirement as conventional amino acid solutions and dialyse as necessary. In some patients electrolyte free solutions may be helpful (see Chapter 6) and for those unable to tolerate a conventional volume load concentrated solutions such as Aminoplex 24 may be useful. The clinical role of solutions of essential amino acids or alpha keto analogues remains to be established.

7.8.3 CHRONIC RENAL FAILURE

Nutritional recommendations have changed following the introduction of dialysis and new ideas about the progression of renal impairment.

(a) Dietary protein

Originally patients were given low protein diets to relieve uraemic symptoms. These restrictions were relaxed during the 1970s when dialysis became widely available. However in the 1980s attention has focused on the potential role of liberal protein diets in the genesis of glomerulosclerosis.

A heavy protein meal increases renal blood flow and glomerular filtration rate, so high protein diets may lead to prolonged glomerular hyperperfusion and hyperfiltration. In animals with ablation of renal tissue the progressive sclerosis of the remaining glomeruli is retarded by protein restriction, and preliminary work suggests that the rate of decline of renal function may be substantially reduced by restricting protein intake in patients with chronic renal failure. Much work is required to determine the role of protein restriction, and in particular the stage at which it should be introduced. However the prospect of deferring or delaying dialysis is of major economic significance.

Traditionally dietary protein restriction is imposed only when the glomerular filtration rate reaches 25 ml/min, with allowances of 70, 50 and 40 g as the filtration rate falls from 25 to 20, 15 and 10 ml/min respectively. Enough protein must be given to prevent wasting, but excess is avoided to prevent the accumulation of nitrogenous waste products, phosphates, sulphates and electrolytes. The minimum needs are 0.5–0.6 g/kg (e.g. 35–40 g per day) which must be delivered as high-quality protein such as eggs and milk which contain a high percentage of essential amino acids. Diets which contain less than 40 g of protein per day are rarely required because of the general availability of dialysis. When used they need supplementation with essential amino acids or their alpha keto analogues. The latter were originally introduced in an attempt to re-utilize waste nitrogen. However they may also be used in patients with moderate protein restriction to increase the range of acceptable dietary protein. The inclusion of protein sources other than those of high biological value makes the diet more varied and interesting.

Additional allowances must be given to patients with nephrotic syndrome and those who are undergoing dialysis. The former require extra protein equivalent to their urinary loss. Patients undergoing haemodialysis need 0.8–1.0 g/kg per day, but greater losses are sustained by peritoneal dialysis and in these patients the basic allowances are doubled. Generally a more liberal diet is permissible in patients who undergo dialysis yet excessive amounts of protein should be avoided.

(b) Energy

The amount of food ingested is normally determined by its energy content. Patients with chronic renal failure must obtain sufficient energy to prevent gluconeogenesis and muscle wasting and enhance protein utilization. This is frequently difficult to achieve because of anorexia and nausea. Conversely excess energy ingestion in the form of both carbohydrate and fat should be avoided because of secondary hypertriglyceridaemia and hypercholesterolaemia. Under these circumstances carbohydrate restriction and the use of polyunsaturated fat may be helpful.

Approximate energy requirements in adults are 30–50 kcal/kg per day (0.13–0.21 MJ), in children they are 50–100 kcal/kg per day (0.21–0.42 MJ).

(c) Minerals

(i) Sodium   Patients may continue to excrete sodium until the creatinine clearance has fallen below 10 ml/min but they are unable to adjust the excretion rapidly with changing intakes. Sudden restriction may risk hypovolaemia and deterioration in renal function. Such patients are able to receive a relatively free diet containing up to 100 mmol of sodium per day. Greater restriction need only apply to hypertensive and oedematous patients, and abrupt reduction in dietary sodium should be avoided. When restriction is required dietary intake can be reduced to 50 mmol per day by avoiding salty foods such as salted crisps and peanuts and by avoiding the addition of salt at the table and in cooking.

Table 7.7 Examples of foods with a high potassium content

Cereals
    Wholegrain breakfast cereals
    Wholemeal and brown bread
    Wholegrain crispbreads
    Oatcakes
Vegetables
    Beans: broad, butter, haricot, baked
    Brussels sprouts, spinach, tomatoes, mushrooms
    Split peas, lentils, leeks
Fruits
    Dried fruits, prunes, dates
    Grapefruit, oranges
Drinks
    Instant coffee, strong tea
    Natural fruit juice, tomato juice
    Oxo, bovril, marmite
Miscellaneous
    Toffee, chocolate, liquorice
    Fruitcake, gingerbread
    Nuts, crisps

(ii) Potassium During conservative management restriction may not be needed until the glomerular filtration rate has fallen below 10 ml/min. Patients undergoing dialysis have lost their ability to excrete potassium and they are allowed more protein in the diet through which more potassium is ingested, so potassium restriction is needed. Such patients are advised to limit their ingestion of foods rich in potassium. Some of these are listed in Table 7.7. Boiled potatoes, boiled rice and pasta are useful substitutes and fruit such as apples and melons are also low in potassium. Ion exchange resins are a helpful adjunct to protein restriction.

(iii) Phosphate As the glomerular filtration rate falls phosphate accumulates and leads to a reciprocal reduction in serum calcium concentration and hence hyperparathyroidism. This further impairs renal function and contributes to renal osteodystrophy.

Dietary phosphate restriction is difficult to achieve. Phosphate is found in protein, particularly in protein of high biological value such as milk and cheese. Large amounts are found in processed foods and carbonated drinks which should be avoided. Consequently phosphate is bound in the gut lumen. Calcium carbonate has replaced aluminium hydroxide for the purpose of phosphate restriction following the incrimination of the latter in the genesis of dialysis dementia and renal osteodystrophy.

(iv) Calcium Protein restriction leads to calcium deficiency. Calcium supplements should be given after the phosphate has been reduced. Calcium carbonate is ideal for this purpose.

(v) Iron and zinc Protein restriction reduces the intake of both these minerals, and iron loss may be enhanced by platelet dysfunction especially in menstruating females. Supplements may be needed particularly in the dialysed patient. Zinc supplementation has been claimed to improve altered taste sensation and appetite.

(d) Vitamins

(i) Folate Patients with chronic renal failure tend to have low serum folate concentrations. Many foods rich in folate such as green vegetables and meat are restricted in these patients, and folate is destroyed by cooking methods used to leach potassium e.g. the soaking and boiling of vegetables. It is also lost during dialysis. A daily supplement of 1 mg is recommended.

(ii) Vitamin C The restriction of fruits and loss through dialysis necessitate a supplement of 50–100 mg per day.

(iii) Pyridoxine Pyridoxine requirements are also increased because of circulating inhibitors, increased metabolic clearance and impaired absorption with drugs such as Hydrallazine which may still be used in some patients. A supplement of 2 mg per day is recommended.

(iv) Vitamin D The metabolism of Vitamin D is impaired with the failure to form the active 1,25 hydroxy Vitamin D from the 25 hydroxy intermediate. Patients should receive 1-alpha Vitamin D or 1,25 hydroxy Vitamin D to prevent renal osteodystrophy.

7.8.4 RENAL CALCULI

The common forms of renal calculi are listed in Table 7.8. With the exception of patients with steatorrhoea there is little evidence to suggest that increased oxalate absorption contributes to the formation of oxalate stones, hence dietary oxalate restriction is not recommended for most patients. A purine free diet is difficult and therefore not used for patients with uric acid calculi. Reduction of dietary

Table 7.8 Common types of renal calculi

Calcium oxalate
Calcium phosphate
Uric acid
Triple phosphate
Cystine

calcium is appropriate when this is excessive as in the milk alkalis syndrome, but excessive restriction will enhance oxalate absorption. Overall dietary manipulation has a negligible role in the management of renal calculus disease.

7.9 Respiratory disease

Abnormal respiratory function and respiratory disease may complicate under-nutrition, discussed here as malnutrition, or obesity. Respiratory disease is often associated with the development of malnutrition. Food allergy has also been incriminated in asthma, and this subject will be discussed in the next chapter.

7.9.1 RESPIRATORY DISEASE AND MALNUTRITION

(a) Pulmonary disorders and malnutrition

Patients with chronic pulmonary disease are often thin and wasted. This particularly applies to those with emphysema, bronchial carcinoma and bronchiectasis. The reason for wasting in emphysematous patients is unclear, but those with carcinoma sometimes suffer from malignant cachexia and patients with bronchiectasis from chronic sepsis.

(b) The effect of malnutrition on respiratory function

Respiratory function depends upon ventilatory drive, the performance of respiratory muscles, and lung function. The primary muscles of inspiration include the diaphragm, internal intercostals and scalene muscles. Malnutrition will impair their performance in three ways.

- During starvation there is a change in muscle geometry with increasing alveolar space and lung volumes. Consequently the diaphragm becomes flatter and shorter and develops less tension
- There is a reduction in muscle mass and thus a decline in strength and endurance
- Malnutrition may be associated with metabolic disorders such as hypophosphataemia, hypomagnesaemia, and hypokalaemia which further impair muscle performance

(c) The effect of nutritional support on respiratory requirements

The metabolism of dextrose, protein and fat provides energy but requires the provision of oxygen and the removal of carbon dioxide as shown in Table 7.9. Patients who are hypermetabolic due to sepsis or

Table 7.9　Energy metabolism and gas exchange

Substrate (1 g)		Oxygen required (ml)		Energy (kcal)		Carbon dioxide (ml)
Carbohydrate	+	829	→	4.1	+	829
Protein	+	966	→	4.1	+	782
Fat	+	2019	→	9.3	+	1427

trauma will have increased nutrient and respiratory demands. More respiratory work can be created by nutrient over-provision. During the infusion of increasing amounts of dextrose into stressed patients an oxidation plateau is observed: a small amount of this difference is accounted for by muscle glycogen formation, the majority by lipo-genesis and increased sympathetic activity. There are large associated increases in carbon dioxide production and oxygen consumption and during lipogenesis the respiratory quotient is greater than one. Nutrition-induced thermogenesis is very high with amino acid solutions and low with lipid. It is similar overall for enteral and parenteral feeding, which means that the cost of digestion and absorption is low in comparison to storage, but it may be greater during bolus feeding due to the increased rate of nutrient storage.

(d) Clinical implications

Three points emerge which are of importance when nutritional support is delivered to malnourished patients who have impaired respiratory function.

- The over-provision of energy and especially nitrogen must be avoided
- Part of the energy should be delivered as lipid
- Refeeding may impose additional respiratory demands before respiratory function improves

Careful attention to these details may reduce the need for, or facilitate weaning from, artificial ventilation.

7.9.2 RESPIRATORY DISEASE AND OBESITY

Obesity impairs respiratory function. Increased abdominal pressure splints the diaphragm and more work is required to move the thicker abdominal wall. In extreme obesity the lung volumes are so changed that the closing volume may encroach on the tidal volume leading to ventilation perfusion inequalities and hypoxaemia. This can ultimately cause pulmonary hypertension and cor pulmonale.

7.10 Haemopoietic diseases

7.10.1 HAEMATINIC DEFICIENCY SYNDROMES

The sources and normal requirements of haematinics are discussed in Chapter 3. Clinical aspects of haematinic deficiency are reviewed in Chapter 4.

(a) Iron

Recommended daily allowances of iron range from 1.5 mg during the first year of life, 10 mg in the adult male, to 18 mg in the adolescent and menstruating female. Dietary sources of iron include liver, red meat, beans, peas and enriched bread. Non-haem iron is absorbed actively in the duodenum and proximal jejunum by a process that is increased in iron deficiency and reduced when stores are sufficient. Absorption is impaired by binding to phytate, phosphate and antacids and is increased by ascorbic acid. Haem iron is absorbed into the enterocyte by a different process. Overall 10% of dietary iron is absorbed.

Iron deficiency is caused by a poor diet, gastrointestinal or excessive menstrual losses. Sometimes more than one cause is found, pregnancy frequently precipitates or aggravates this syndrome. Gastrointestinal losses in this country are usually attributable to malabsorption or bleeding from ulcers, cancers or inflammatory bowel disease. Universally worm infestation and poor diet are the most important problems leading to iron deficiency.

The hallmark of iron deficiency is a microcytic hypochromic blood film. The patient may complain of tiredness, symptoms secondary to the cardiovascular effects of anaemia such as angina or dyspnoea, or symptoms of the underlying disease. Angular cheilitis and koilonychia are occasional features. In addition to treating any underlying disease dietary advice and iron supplements usually restore the haemoglobin and alleviate symptoms.

(b) Folate

Most patients require 200 μg, the recommended daily allowance is 400 μg, with 800 μg in pregnancy and 1 mg after dialysis. Folate is found in liver, green vegetables, nuts, and yeast. It is absorbed in the proximal small bowel.

Folate deficiency is caused by a poor diet or by inappropriate methods of food preparation such as over-cooking vegetables. There is impaired absorption in patients with gluten enteropathy and alcohol addiction. Increased requirements or losses occur in pregnancy, haemodialysis and haemolytic anaemia.

Deficiency causes impaired nucleic acid and amino acid synthesis, and the major impact occurs in cells with rapid turnover such as the bone marrow and intestinal epithelium. The patient will exhibit general features of anaemia and possibly glossitis, though dementia is a rare feature. The diagnosis is suggested by the finding of a macrocytic anaemia with nuclear hypersegmentation.

(c) Vitamin B12

The recommended daily intake is 2 μg, with 4 μg during pregnancy and lactation. Most patients have relatively large stores of 2–3 mg mostly in the liver. Consequently there is a long latent period between reduced intake and clinical presentation. Sources of Vitamin B12 include liver, red meat, milk, and cheese. Absorption occurs by active transport in the terminal ileum following combination with intrinsic factor secreted by the gastric mucosa.

Deficiency of Vitamin B12 may be dietary. Most vegetarians eat animal produce such as milk or cheese and consequently receive adequate supplies, but vegans take no animal produce whatsoever. Nevertheless deficiency is not universal among such people presumably because of food contamination by yeast or synthesis by micro-organisms. More commonly deficiency occurs due to loss of intrinsic factor in pernicious anaemia or following gastric surgery, disruption of the intrinsic factor complex in the bowel lumen by bacterial colonization or fish tapeworm, or loss of terminal ileal function in Crohn's disease or after bowel resection. Rarely it may be congenital due to transcobalamine II deficiency.

Patients develop a megaloblastic anaemia with macrocytosis and polymorphonuclear hyperpigmentation, and they may also be icteric due to ineffective erythropoiesis. Glossitis may occur. However the most serious potential impact is in the central nervous system. Peripheral neuropathy, sub-acute combined degeneration of the cord and dementia may develop, and the central effects may not be reversible.

Most patients need parenteral replacement. Oral supplementation can be used for those with dietary deficiency.

(d) Miscellaneous haematinics

Pyridoxine deficiency will lead to a hypochromic microcytic anaemia. Vitamin E deficiency is characterized by a haemolytic anaemia. These deficiencies occur rarely and usually in the context of obvious malnutrition.

7.10.2 HAEMOLYTIC ANAEMIA

Haemolytic anaemias may be congenital due to an abnormality of the red cell haemoglobin or acquired due to auto-immune disease or drug therapy. Loss of folate necessitates supplementation in such patients.

7.10.3 HAEMATOLOGICAL MALIGNANCY

The treatment of leukaemia by intense chemotherapy damages tissues particularly those with rapid cell turnover such as the bone marrow and intestinal mucosa. These drugs also lead to protracted vomiting. Thus parenteral nutrition may be needed to maintain nutritional status during this type of treatment.

7.11 Diseases of bone

7.11.1 OSTEOPOROSIS

Osteoporosis is a reduction in bone mass the composition of which is normal. Patients are prone to fractures of long bones for example fracture of the neck of femur and Colles fracture, or of vertebral bodies.

(a) Causes of osteoporosis

Bone mass declines with age in everyone but the initial bone mass and the rate of decline vary. Loss of bone is much more rapid in post-menopausal women so osteoporosis occurs more commonly in elderly females. Idiopathic osteoporosis affects younger patients. Known causes of osteoporosis include corticosteroid excess, hyperthyroidism or hypogonadism, and it affects patients who are immobile. In malabsorptive states osteoporosis is frequently associated with osteomalacia.

(b) The diet and osteoporosis

Dietary calcium deficiency is of importance in the development of osteoporosis. This will induce osteoporosis in animals but the evidence is less convincing in humans. A difficulty arises because many foods affect the utilization of calcium. Calcium absorption is reduced by phosphates, oxalates (green vegetables), phytates (unleavened bread) as well as by a high intraluminal fat content and Vitamin D deficiency. Consequently dietary calcium has to be considered in relation to other nutrients especially phosphate.

The optimum ratio of calcium to phosphate is 1:1 and the recommended daily allowance of each is 800 mg. Even with low calcium diets the patient may remain in balance provided the dietary phosphate is correspondingly low. Conversely high calcium diets may not necessarily protect against osteoporosis if the dietary phosphate content is even greater because of impaired absorption. Foods which contain more phosphate than calcium include meat, poultry and fish and a high protein diet may have a calcuric effect because of the enhanced excretion of sulphate. Milk, natural cheese and leaf vegetables contain more calcium than phosphate. Unfortunately phosphate is an additive in food processing and is found in soft drinks and processed cheese.

The nutritional implications are clear. The diet should provide the recommended allowance of calcium, and additional calcium may be necessary if there is a high phosphate content and in the elderly in whom calcium absorption can be impaired. Prophylaxis is much more effective than treatment, since additional calcium may retard the development of osteoporosis but it will not restore lost bone.

(c) Osteoporosis and parenteral nutrition

Osteoporosis appears to be a problem in patients who undergo long-term cyclical parenteral feeding as opposed to continuous intravenous feeding. There is evidence that intermittent and thus more rapid infusion induces the negative calcium balance, possibly because of increased buffering requirements. The advantages of cyclical feeding in terms of patient mobility, water and fat retention and home parenteral nutrition are obvious. This finding is a cause for concern.

7.11.2 OSTEOMALACIA

Osteomalacia results from a lack of Vitamin D and is characterized by defective bone mineralization. The clinical features of Vitamin D deficiency are described in Chapter 4. They include rickets in children, bone pain and myopathy in adults.

(a) Causes of osteomalacia

Causes of osteomalacia include the inadequate supply of Vitamin D because of a diet lacking in oily fish, dairy produce and liver, combined with inadequate exposure to the sun. The elderly and immigrant populations are particularly susceptible to this problem.

Patients with intestinal, pancreatic and cholestatic disease absorb vitamins poorly, and those with renal failure may fail to metabolize the active 1,25 hydroxy Vitamin D from 25 hydroxy Vitamin D formed in the liver. In epileptics and alcoholics enzyme induction leads to an increased degradation of the active metabolite.

(b) Management of osteomalacia

Patients with dietary deficiency who have developed osteomalacia require supplements of 2000–4000 units of Vitamin D a day for three months. Thereafter recurrent disease can be prevented either by a maintenance dose of 200–400 units a day or by eating an adequate diet containing sufficient supplies of vitamins. Patients with malabsorption will require larger doses and parenteral administration e.g. 600 000 units of calciferol a year. Careful monitoring is needed to prevent overdosage and subsequent hypercalcaemia. The active metabolite in the form of 1,25 hydroxy Vitamin D or 1-alpha Vitamin D is needed by patients with renal failure. An additional advantage of these compounds is their short half life and reduced risk of significant hypercalcaemia.

7.12 Neurological disease

7.12.1 CEREBROVASCULAR DISEASE

Cerebrovascular disease is very common, and mortality and morbidity are greater than for ischaemic heart disease. It is strongly associated with hypertension and many of these patients are obese. Nutritional factors in the genesis of vascular disease are discussed in Sections 7.6 and 7.7.

The nutritional implications of a stroke are considerable. Many patients are depressed and do not wish to eat. A negative nitrogen balance can have unfavourable effects on residual muscle function, impairing mobilization. Some patients are unable to feed themselves and require careful assistance. Swallowing is difficult and often temporarily impossible in the case of bulbar or pseudo-bulbar palsy. Naso-gastric feeding by fine bore tube is very useful under these circumstances.

A significant number of patients are obese, which may be a contributory factor in the pathogenesis of their stroke and makes mobilization more difficult. These patients need dietetic supervision. This also applies to diabetic patients who are particularly prone to vascular disease. Consequently expert dietetic care is frequently required.

7.12.2 MULTIPLE SCLEROSIS

This is a disease which affects one in 2000 people in Britain. It is characterized by areas of demyelination in the central nervous system, relapses and remissions, and a tendency to increasing neurological disability with diplopia, weakness and unco-ordinated movement.

The cause of multiple sclerosis is unknown: both slow virus infection and immunological disorder have been postulated. The observation that a similar pathological process in sheep is associated with a loss of cerebral lecithins in which the saturated-to-unsaturated fatty acid ratio is increased, and that human sufferers have a reduced linoleic acid concentration in plasma and phospholipids of red cell membranes, prompted a trial of linoleic acid given as sunflower seed oil emulsion. Sadly initial enthusiasm has not been justified by clinical trials, although many patients still receive these supplements.

As the patient's mobility is reduced so it is necessary to reduce the energy content of the diet. Failure to do so will lead to obesity. Obesity will prematurely curtail mobility and increase nursing difficulties. In the latter stages of disease naso-gastric feeding may be helpful.

7.12.3 EPILEPSY

Epilepsy is common and affects one in 200 of the population. Most epileptics are readily controlled by drugs. Some of these for example Phenytoin and Phenobarbitone induce microsomal enzymes and predispose to osteomalacia by enhancing metabolism of 1,25 hydroxy Vitamin D. Folate deficiency also occurs for the same reason. Epileptic patients should avoid alcohol which potentiates the epileptic tendency.

Children with epilepsy who do not respond to anticonvulsant drugs occasionally benefit from a ketogenic diet. Although rarely needed it appears particularly helpful in childhood myoclonic epilepsy. Medium chain triglyceride oil is used to provide 60–70% of the energy requirements. Disadvantages include offensive diarrhoea and possible reduction in growth rate. There is no evidence that such a diet predisposes to cardiovascular disease.

7.12.4 MIGRAINE

Classical migraine is characterized by a severe unilateral headache often preceded by a visual aura and accompanied by photophoia and vomiting. There have been claims that attacks are provoked by factors in the diet: chocolate and cheese have been cited in this context. The subject of food intolerance is discussed in the next chapter.

7.12.5 HYPERACTIVITY

This term is applied to children whose behaviour is abnormal and disruptive. They are hyperactive, impulsive, frequently aggressive and have difficulty in concentrating. Many are brain damaged. Some of these children respond to the withdrawal of food additives especially colouring agents such as tartrazine.

7.12.6 MOTOR NEURONE DISEASE

Motor neurone disease is a devastating degenerative disorder of unknown cause which leads to progressive motor failure often with a combination of upper and lower motor neurone features. Bulbar and pseudo-bulbar palsy make swallowing difficult, so naso-gastric feeding may be helpful.

7.13 Obesity

7.13.1 DEFINITION OF OBESITY

Obesity refers to the excessive accumulation of fat which is known to be associated with excess morbidity and mortality. Satisfactory clinical methods for the reliable measurement of fat are not available, so body weight has been used as an index of adiposity. For a long time

Table 7.10 The optimum range of body weight for height: taken from the 1979 Fogarty Conference

Males Height (cm)	Acceptable weight (kg)	Overweight (kg)	Obese (kg)
158	44–64	70	77
162	46–66	73	79
166	48–69	76	83
170	51–73	80	88
174	53–75	83	90
178	55–79	87	95
182	59–82	90	98
186	62–86	95	103
190	66–90	99	108

Females Height (cm)	Acceptable weight (kg)	Overweight (kg)	Obese (kg)
150	38–55	61	66
154	39–57	63	68
158	40–58	64	70
162	42–61	67	73
166	44–64	70	77
170	45–66	73	79
174	48–69	76	83
178	51–72	79	86

acceptable weight has been considered in relation to frame size, but unfortunately no precise definition of frame size exists. Measurements can be simplified using the Quetelet or body mass index of w/h^2 where w = weight in kg and h = height in metres. By this method the index of weights at different heights is found to be the same. Using this index the values associated with the lowest mortality have been determined and thus a range of acceptable weights for each height calculated. These acceptable ranges are taken from the 1979 USA Fogarty Conference and are shown in Table 7.10.

Many authorities define overweight and obesity as weights which are 10% and 20% above the upper limits of this range. Clearly this index takes no account of the relative contribution of muscle mass and adipose tissue. One clinical method of estimating the latter uses skin fold thickness measured by Harpenden calipers. The method of skin fold thickness measurement is discussed in Chapter 4. The normal sum of the four standard skin folds is 40 mm: measurements of 60 mm and 80 mm correlate with the above definitions of overweight and obesity. In most patients obesity can be diagnosed on clinical inspection, and such refinements are normally only required for epidemiological surveys.

7.13.2 THE PATHOGENESIS OF OBESITY

Secondary obesity is rare. It may be caused by damage to the hypothalamus, endocrine disorders such as hypothyroidism or Cushing's syndrome, enforced inactivity, or drugs including corticosteroids, anabolic agents and sulphonylureas. Most obesity is primary, arising from both genetic and environmental influences.

The three major factors which have been considered in relation to the development of obesity are food intake, physical activity and thermogenesis.

(a) Energy intake

Claims that obese patients eat more than their lean counterparts have not always been substantiated. Under these circumstances previous dietary excesses are blamed for current obesity. However this explanation is unsatisfactory given the knowledge that normal people can maintain their weight within relatively narrow limits in spite of large and varying dietary intakes.

(b) Physical activity

Whereas mobility may be reduced in the obese this can be a consequence of obesity and the energy required for a given activity is greater than in the normal weight individual.

(c) Thermogenesis

Evidence has been presented that some of these patients have a reduced thermogenic response. They are thus metabolically more efficient in terms of energy utilization but are unable to burn off excess nutrients. This is a controversial concept, but if correct it implies the need for lifelong dietary restriction even after excessive weight has been lost.

7.13.3 CLINICAL ASSOCIATIONS OF OBESITY

The diseases with an increased prevalance in obese patients are listed in Table 7.11. Many of these patients are in a pre-diabetic state with reduced glucose tolerance and hyperinsulinaemia which may reflect reduced numbers of insulin receptors. Ketone body production is

Table 7.11 Diseases associated with obesity

Diabetes mellitus
Hypertension
Coronary heart disease
Cholelithiasis
Osteoarthrosis
Gout
Pulmonary disease
Neoplastic disease
Hernias
Varicose veins
Intertrigo

reduced in starvation. Blood cholesterol values are higher in the obese and there is a clear relationship between obesity and hypertension. The risk of coronary heart disease in this group is controversial, since the increased incidence may largely be accounted for by the previous risk factors of diabetes and hypertension. Increased biliary cholesterol secretion predisposes to cholelithiasis and excess weight to osteo-arthrosis. Mechanical factors associated with increased abdominal pressure contribute to the development of hernias, varicose veins, and impaired respiratory function. The latter is discussed in Section 7.9.

7.13.4 THE TREATMENT OF OBESITY

(a) General management

Causes of secondary obesity must be excluded or where present treated. Underlying psychological factors should be explored and when depression or anxiety contributes to an abnormal eating pattern specific management is required. The patient needs educating not only with reference to the detrimental effect of obesity on health but to the underlying principles involved in weight reduction.

(b) Dietary management

The induction of a negative energy balance and the subsequent prevention of weight gain is the basis of treatment. Patients must be told that one kilogram weight loss corresponds to a negative balance of 7700 kcal (32 MJ) from adipose stores and consequently the rate of weight loss will be slow, approximately one kilogram a week using conventional diets. Many patients are encouraged by the initial rapid weight loss that accompanies mobilization of glycogen and muscle protein: both are in an aqueous phase and their metabolism is accompanied by fluid loss. They become despondent when metabolic adaption leads to fat mobilization and slow weight loss.

Most diets provide 1000 kcal (4.2 MJ) less than the estimated requirements. Women are advised to eat 800–1000 kcal (4.2 MJ) and men 1200–1500 kcal (6.3 MJ). Traditionally this was achieved by carbohydrate restriction but the increased consumption of fat is no longer acceptable. It is better to advise patients about the calorie content of foods. Three meals should be eaten daily, 'empty' calories in the form of refined carbohydrate, alcohol or fat should be avoided or reduced, and nibbling between meals forbidden. Increasing the time spent over meals and the consumption of high fibre supplements both increases satiety and reduces the temptation to over-eat.

For non–compliant patients total starvation used to be employed on an in-patient basis. Nitrogen loss and death from cardiac dysrhythmia associated with electrolyte imbalance now prohibits such an approach. This led to the introduction of specially formulated liquid diets which provide up to 400 kcal with limited fat, around 40 g of protein containing the required essential amino acids, and the recommended allowance of micronutrients. Examples include Modifast, Uni-Vite, and the Cambridge Diet. These preparations will enhance weight loss, particularly in obese women with low metabolic rates for whom a conventional yet nutritionally complete diet may be difficult to prescribe. They should only be used for limited periods under supervision and they make no contribution to the re-education of eating habits. Additional bulking agents are sometimes needed to overcome constipation.

(c) Other forms of management

Drugs are frequently prescribed but are of limited value. Fenfluramine is the most commonly used as an appetite suppressant. This may have a role early in treatment to help the patient comply with the diet. Some centres have used it intermittently on an alternate month basis. Caffeine is the most widely used drug that enhances thermogenesis. At present the safety and place of tri-iodothyramine are not established and it should not be used.

Reputable commercial slimming organizations give valuable support and encouragement to many patients. Some clinicians employ the clinical psychologist in a programme of behaviour modification. This is particularly aimed at the person who continually nibbles between meals or who resorts to food to relieve underlying tensions.

Many surgical approaches have been devised to reduce nutrient intake or absorption. Jaw wiring prevents the consumption of solid foods. It requires careful dental supervision to prevent dental caries, inhalation is a risk in patients who are prone to vomit, and high calorie liquids are readily found. Currently gastric banding or plication is gaining popularity as a way of reducing the size of the gastric pouch and enhancing early satiety, though ischaemic perforation is an uncommon technical hazard. The endoscopic placement of an inflatable balloon has been used to achieve the same purpose but requires further evaluation. The same applies to truncal vagotomy. Jejuno-ileal bypass surgery is no longer acceptable because it leads to complications, particularly liver disease.

The recent introduction of a nylon abdominal band which can be tightened but not slackened is an interesting concept to encourage dietary compliance. If the patient over-eats the band becomes tight, and eventually it may have to be cut. As the compliant patient loses weight it is progressively adjusted.

7.14 Anorexia nervosa and bulimia nervosa

7.14.1 ANOREXIA NERVOSA

This is an increasingly common condition with a prevalence of 1% in a schoolgirl population of 16–18 years. It is characterized by abnormal attitudes about weight and shape, considerable self-induced weight loss, and amenorrhoea. Half of these patients have a previous history of being overweight.

Patients with anorexia nervosa are secretive about eating and eat small meals very slowly, avoiding foods of high calorie density. They can be very devious and food is frequently hidden or discarded. Occasional episodes of bulimia occur. Subsequent attempts to dispose of food involve self-induced vomiting and the abuse of purgatives and diuretics. Thus in addition to weight loss which can result in severe malnutrition electrolyte imbalance especially hypokalaemia may develop.

Nutritional management involves the correction of specific nutrient deficiencies such as potassium and iron, and encouraging the patient to re-establish a normal eating pattern. When the patient is grossly emaciated a light diet of about 1500 kcal (6.3 MJ) should be administered in small aliquots at 2-hourly intervals to reduce the risk of problems such as gastric dilatation or perforation and paralytic ileus. Subsequently the diet is gradually increased and presented as normal but attractive meals of up to 4000 kcal (16.8 MJ). Patient compliance is encouraged by a system of rewards and monitored by weight.

Initially there may be a considerable weight increase due to water retention. This is followed by a period in which there is no weight gain or even weight loss. Thereafter weight should be gained at a rate of 1.5 kg a week.

Occasionally parenteral nutrition is needed for patients who are difficult to manage, severely emaciated or who develop intestinal complications such as paralytic ileus or gastric dilatation. However the oral route should be employed as soon as possible and the pattern of regular meals in the company of other people established at an early stage.

7.14.2 PARTIAL SYNDROME

Subclinical anorexia nervosa is common. Patients are distinguished from the customary dieter by a preoccupation with weight and shape and a drive to obtain an unrealistically low ideal weight. Most do not develop the full spectrum of the anorexic syndrome.

7.14.3 BULIMIA AND BULIMIA NERVOSA

In literature from the USA bulimia is described as a syndrome characterized by recurrent episodes of compulsive binge eating with or without self-induced vomiting or purgation. Bulimia nervosa is also a binge eating syndrome in which there is induced vomiting and a fear of fatness. The overlap with anorexia nervosa is obvious. Electrolyte imbalance occurs in this disorder but it is not associated with gross nutritional depletion.

7.15 Cancer

Patients with malignant disease frequently lose weight and appear malnourished or emaciated. Nutritional interest has focused on two areas: the effect of the tumour on the nutritional state of a patient, and the effect of nutritional support on the tumour growth. The degree of wasting and weight loss bears no relation to the tumour size or type and is probably multifactorial in origin.

7.15.1 CAUSES OF CACHEXIA

Many patients with cancer reduce their food intake. The reasons may be mechanical in those with gastro-oesophageal or intestinal tumours, but more commonly other mechanisms operate. Altered taste sensation, depression, pain, nausea, hypercalcaemia and drugs individually or collectively depress the appetite.

Malabsorption has been documented in some tumours which appear to cause morphological change in the small intestine. The small intestine is particularly sensitive to cytotoxic chemotherapy. Blood protein or other nutrients may be lost through the bowel or into the peritoneal or pleural cavities via malignant ulceration.

In contrast to starvation the basal metabolic rate is increased. Host-metabolism may be altered, and tumours which tend to be glycolytic produce lactate which is recycled to glucose by gluconeogenesis in the liver (Cori cycle: see Chapter 2), an inefficient process which uses energy. The production of toxic tumour substrates may also be important and it has been suggested that tumours utilize substrate at the expense of the host.

7.15.2 CONSEQUENCES OF CACHEXIA

Typically the patient feels weak and tired. Cachexia has a detrimental effect on the quality of life, predisposes the patient to infection, delays wound healing, and enhances operative risk.

7.15.3 NUTRITIONAL MANAGEMENT

Correction of hypercalcaemia, pain control, and allowance for altered taste sensation will often permit an improved oral diet. Many of these patients are nauseated by sweet foods and prefer savoury flavours. Dietary supplements and whole protein polymeric diets are now available in a range of flavours the prescription of which should be tailored to the individual patient. Naso-gastric feeding may be useful in weak patients with profound anorexia. Those with intestinal failure or intestinal obstruction will require parenteral nutrition. However this should only be used when there is a significant prospect of recovery or at least partial remission.

Patients may be categorized into two groups according to their response to nutritional support. Those in whom nutrition has been inadequate for mechanical reasons or due to anorexia e.g. with oesophageal or gastric carcinoma may benefit from a period of nutritional repletion before undergoing definitive surgery. Many patients however fail to respond even to aggressive hyperalimentation unless the offending tumour can be treated or removed. A prolonged period of pre-operative nutritional support in this group is not appropriate.

7.15.4 NUTRITIONAL SUPPORT AND TUMOUR GROWTH

The fear that nutritional support would preferentially feed the tumour and hasten its growth at the expense of the host has not been substantiated. Neither has the hope that nutritional support would significantly improve the host tolerance of more aggressive chemotherapeutic regimes and thereby improve treatment outcome. This is a grey area which has been extensively studied with inconclusive results.

7.16 Inborn errors of metabolism

Detailed description of this complex subject is beyond the scope of this book. Discussion will be confined to a summary of a limited number of metabolic defects in which diet plays an important part in management.

7.16.1 DISORDERS OF AROMATIC AMINO ACIDS

(a) Hyperphenylalanaemia (phenylketonuria)

Impaired hydroxylation of phenylalanine to tyrosine leads to hyperphenylalanaemia. Several types have been recognized. Clinical features include mental retardation, microcephaly, fits and abnormal skin pigmentation.

Treatment aims to keep the plasma concentration of phenylalanine within the range 0.18–0.49 mmol/l. This is achieved with a diet reduced in phenylalanine based on a synthetic substitute for most dietary protein. At one month the baby may only tolerate the minimum protein requirement of 70–90 mg/kg, but the diet becomes easier by the second year when the minimum requirement is reduced to 35 mg/kg. Over-treatment is to be avoided because phenylalanine deficiency also leads to mental deficiency, rashes, hair loss and failure to thrive.

Tolerance of phenylalanine may change during childhood, and periodic assessment by phenylalanine challenge is useful. Traditionally the diet is stopped by the age of eight years when the period of maximum susceptibility to brain damage has passed. Nevertheless consumption of first-class protein should be restricted to keep phenylalanine levels below 1.82 mmol/l. Furthermore there is some evidence that more prolonged restriction may aid subsequent development and some authorities consider that females should remain on the diet until they have passed child-bearing age.

(b) Tyrosinaemia type 1

Tyrosine is derived from the diet or by the hydroxylation of phenylalanine. Clinical features of this disorder include hepatosplenomegaly with haemolytic anaemia and cirrhosis. The Fanconi syndrome is common.

Treatment involves the restriction of tyrosine. Phenylalanine and methionine should be controlled by monitoring the blood values. Large doses of Vitamin D are required because of the Fanconi syndrome. Most patients die of hepatic failure.

7.16.2 UREA CYCLE DISORDERS

Several metabolic defects of the urea cycle enzymes lead to hyperammonaemia with clinical features of vomiting, episodic confusion, ataxia, altered behaviour, and mental handicap. Surprisingly the blood urea tends to be normal.

Dietary management involves protein restriction from birth, allowing sufficient protein for growth e.g. 1–1.5 g/kg in infancy. Arginine supplements should be prescribed because of a reduced synthesis of this amino acid. The use of alpha keto analogues of essential amino acids as a means of reducing ammonia production, particularly during intercurrent infections, is under evaluation.

7.16.3 BRANCH CHAIN AMINO ACID DISORDERS

Branch chain amino acids (leucine, isoleucine, and valine) are transaminated to the corresponding alpha oxoacids. Defective oxidative decarboxylation of these gives rise to maple syrup urine disease. The classical disease causes death or severe brain damage in the neonatal period, when high leucine concentrations lead to hypoglycaemia. There also exists a milder form of disease and an intermittent type precipitated by infection.

Restriction of dietary branch chain amino acids from an early age has been beneficial. Protein may have to be withdrawn during periods of acute infection. The necessary duration of such management is not known.

7.16.4 ERRORS OF METABOLISM OF SULPHUR-CONTAINING AMINO ACIDS

In patients with homocystinurea, cystathione synthase deficiency leads to an accumulation of homocysteine which is oxidized to homocystine. Patients are tall with high arched palates and arachnodactyl. Lens dislocation, optic atrophy and thromboembolism are common, and half are mentally retarded. Biochemical abnormalities can be reduced by restricting methionine and giving cystine with pharmacological doses of pyridoxine.

7.17 Intensive care

Many patients who receive intensive care are seriously ill. They have trauma, sepsis or burns with respiratory, cardiac or renal impairment. Some have multi-system failure and in the majority gastrointestinal function is impaired and intestinal ileus is common. No patient in this category can feed by the oral route: naso-gastric or fine bore jejun-ostomy feeding is possible in some, but most need parenteral nutrition.

The first priority is to treat electrolyte, cardiovascular and res-piratory impairment. Circulatory volume must be restored using the appropriate colloid or crystalloid infusion and patients with established or impending respiratory failure will need artificial ventilation. Those with renal failure require dialysis. At this stage attention can be directed to nutritional support.

7.17.1 NUTRITIONAL OBJECTIVES

During the flow phase of injury, restoration of nutritional status and muscle mass cannot be achieved. Metabolism during stress and injury is discussed in Chapter 2. The provision of adequate nutrition will reduce muscle wasting and facilitate tissue healing. However the traditional approach to aggressive hyperalimentation (the supply of excess energy and nitrogen) in which the prescription of up to 5000 kcal (21 MJ) used to be common, is harmful. Not only does it fail to promote muscle synthesis but it stimulates lipogenesis and thus increases carbon dioxide production and oxygen consumption with detrimental effects on gas exchange. It increases thermogenesis with enhanced catecholamine secretion and further stimulation of the catabolic process. The nutritional objectives are thus to conserve the patient and facilitate healing.

7.17.2 METHODS OF FEEDING

The majority of patients are unable to eat. Those in whom the intestine is accessible and functional should receive enteral feeding. The available enteral feeds are discussed in Chapter 5. High energy and nitrogen preparations may be useful e.g. Ensure Twocal. Special enteral formulations are available for patients with respiratory, renal and hepatic failure. Pulmacare has a high fat/low carbohydrate content the significance of which will be discussed below, Nephro-nutril is enriched with essential amino acids and Hepatomine with branch chain amino acids. The clinical value of these preparations requires verification by further study. Traditionally enteral feeds are introduced with starter regimes which involve increments of reducing dilutions and increasing volumes, and this gradual introduction is claimed to prevent diarrhoea. Such methods lead to a significant early negative nitrogen balance and may not be necessary. Diarrhoea is frequently attributable to concomitant drug administration, especially antibiotics.

The majority of patients need parenteral nutrition. Their nutrient requirements and duration of treatment are such that peripheral feeding is impractical. Continuous central parenteral nutrition will be needed for unstable and hypercatabolic patients although cyclical feeding can be introduced as they improve. Careful attention should be paid to nutrient provision.

7.17.3 ENERGY SOURCES

(a) Dextrose and lipid

As discussed previously the capacity to metabolize dextrose is limited on stressed patients to 6 mg/kg per minute. Providing more dextrose will stimulate lipogenesis and thermogenesis. It therefore follows that at least 25% of the energy supply should be delivered as lipid in order to meet possible energy requirements of 40–50 kcal per kg. Many clinicians prefer to provide 50% of the non-protein energy with lipid, provided lipid tolerance has been established and the manufacturers' recommendations are not exceeded. The thermogenic response to lipid is minimal. In the majority of patients with malnutrition and/or moderate catabolism lipid is as effective as dextrose in protein conservation, but this may not apply in those who are severely hypercatabolic with burns.

(b) Insulin

Glucose intolerance and insulin resistance is a feature of the neuro-endocrine response to severe illness and many patients become hyperglycaemic and require insulin to prevent hyperosmolar dehydration.

The use of insulin has been routinely advocated in hypercatabolic patients because it causes additional protein sparing. Furthermore it will reduce hyperkalaemia in patients with renal failure. Conversely insulin may prevent the mobilization of essential fatty acids as well as amino acids from visceral protein. This can be of importance in patients who do not receive lipid and because of the incomplete amino acid spectrum currently available from nitrogen sources. Insulin may increase dextrose-induced thermogenesis.

It is our policy to use insulin only to control hyperglycaemia. Such insulin requirements are initially met by separate infusion and adjusted to keep the blood glucose in the acceptable range of 6–10 mmol/l. Thereafter when the patient has become stable insulin can be added to the nutrient solution.

7.17.4 NITROGEN SOURCE

These patients frequently require 0.3 g of nitrogen per kilogram. Excessive amino acid administration should be avoided, as amino acids are more thermogenic than dextrose. Concentrated solutions such as Aminoplex 24 may be useful in patients who are intolerant of large fluid volumes, and electrolyte-free preparations have a limited use in some patients. Branch chain amino acid solutions may be of value for the management of encephalopathic patients with liver failure, but their role in the prevention of protein wasting in hypercatabolic patients is controversial.

7.18 Nutrition in miscellaneous disorders

7.18.1 CYSTIC FIBROSIS

This is a genetic disease which affects one in 2000 of the population. It is characterized by abnormal exocrine secretions which have increased protein and electrolyte content and increased viscosity. The high sodium concentration in sweat is used in diagnosis. These secretions impair the function of many organs, especially the lungs, pancreas, liver, and intestine. Presentation may occur in the neonatal period with intestinal obstruction due to meconium ileus. Subsequently respiratory disease with infections, bronchiectasis and fibrosis dominates, but severe malabsorption due to exocrine pancreatic insufficiency, cholestasis and intestinal disease leads to malnutrition which can further impair respiratory function and thwart growth.

Specific management of this condition involves physiotherapy, antibiotics, and pancreatic supplements with H_2 antagonists. Nutritional management is particularly important to reverse under-nutrition without aggravating intestinal symptoms.

Patients should receive expert dietetic advice. A high energy and protein diet is required, and 120% of the normal dietary allowance is usually recommended. Fat restriction may reduce steatorrhoea when carbohydrate supplements are needed to maintain energy intake. This can be very difficult with severe fat restriction, so more liberal fat allowances are now given. Some patients tolerate medium chain triglycerides which can be provided as cooking oil or in polymeric enteral feeds. It may be necessary to replace fat soluble vitamins. Sodium depletion due to excessive loss through sweat occasionally requires salt supplements in the pyrexial patient or in hot climates.

Increasingly clinicians are employing an aggressive approach to nutritional support in these patients. Nocturnal naso-gastric hyperalimentation (see Chapter 5) and supplemental parenteral feeding can be very effective in restoring nutritional status and the patient's general welfare.

7.18.2 ACQUIRED IMMUNE DEFICIENCY SYNDROME

The association of chronic diarrhoea with malabsorption and weight loss with immune deficiency states is well known. An increasing number of patients are developing Acquired Immune Deficiency Syndrome and presenting with symptoms of malabsorption. This may be related to infections such as cryptosporidia, cytomegalo virus, giardia lamblia, or mycobacterium avian intracellulare. Some have small intestinal bacterial over-growth and others extensive intestinal involvement with Kaposi's sarcoma. The impact of malabsorption is compounded by enhanced nutritional requirements due to lymphomas or other opportunist infections. Malnutrition is thus a common feature.

Nutritional support by the oral or enteral routes may be needed. Claims that improved nutritional status enhances immune competence in this population require further study.

7.18.3 DISEASES OF THE JOINTS

The role of food antigens in the formation of immune complexes and the development of inflammatory arthritis is speculative and not established. Obesity is associated with degenerative osteoarthrosis of the knees and hips. Such joint disease will limit mobility and indirectly increase obesity.

7.18.4 PSYCHIATRIC DISORDERS

Depression is associated with anorexia and weight loss. Depressed patients, particularly those who live alone, may not bother to prepare meals or eat. Malnutrition is a feature of this disease. Nutritional management is not usually required, as the diet improves with treatment of the depression. It must not be forgotton that patients with protein energy malnutrition appear withdrawn and retarded. Many of these are mistakenly diagnosed as being depressed.

Vanadium-restricted diets have been found to help patients with some types of schizophrenia. This form of management is currently under evaluation. The importance of a high carbohydrate diet in acute attacks of porphyria has previously been emphasized. Carbohydrate suppresses enzyme activity and reduces the synthesis of porphyrins.

7.18.5 NUTRITION AND DERMATOLOGICAL DISEASE

In atopic patients IgE mediated food allergy may present as a contact or generalized urticaria. Foods commonly responsible include eggs, milk, fish, nuts, and strawberries. Urticaria can also develop through non-allergic mechanisms. Chemicals such as tartrazine, benzoates and salicylates, which are either food additives or present in trace amounts in some foods, occasionally release histamine through prostaglandin metabolism. Such patients can benefit from additive-free diets, which are discussed in Chapter 8. The role of food allergy in atopic eczema, as with asthma, is more difficult to define. Occasionally the use of an elimination diet is helpful. Nickel dermatitis is common and may be aggravated by nickel ingestion as a contaminant from cooking-utensils.

Important changes can be seen in the skin in patients who suffer severe malnutrition. These are discussed in Chapter 4.

References

Askanazi, J., Rosenbaum, S. H., Hyman, A. I., Silverberg, P. A., Milie-Emili, J., and Kinney, J. M. (1980) Respiratory changes induced by large glucose loads of total parenteral nutrition. *Journal of the American Medical Association*, **243**, 1444–7.

Baird, J. D. (1982) Diet and diabetes mellitus, in *Nutrition and Health*. Turner, M.R. (ed.), M.T.P. Press Ltd, ch. 10, 135–49.

Brennan, M. F. (1981). Total parenteral nutrition in the cancer patient. *New England Journal of Medicine*, **305**, 375–82.

Brodribb, A. J. M. (1982). Diverticular disease and diet, in *Nutrition and Health*. Turner, M. R. (ed.), M.T.P. Press Ltd, ch. 5, 57–70.

Cooke, W. T. and Holmes, R. (1984). *Coeliac Disease*, Churchill Livingstone, Edinburgh.

De Bruizn, K. M., Blendis, L. M., Zilm, D. H., Carlen, P. L., and Anderson, G. H. (1983) Effect of dietary protein manipulations in subclinical portal-systemic encephalopathy. *Gut*, **24**, 53–60.

El Nahas, A. M. and Coles, G. A. (1986) Dietary treatment of chronic renal failure: ten unanswered questions. *Lancet*, **i**, 597–600.

Fairburn, C. G. (1983) Bulimia nervosa. *British Journal of Hospital Medicine*, **33**, 537–42.

Goodchild, M. C. (1986) Practical management of nutrition and gastro-intestinal tract in cystic fibrosis. *Journal of the Royal Society of Medicine, Supplement 12*, **77**, 32–7.

Halliday, M. A., McHenry-Richardson, K., and Partale, A. (1979). Nutritional management of chronic renal disease. *Medical Clinics of North America*, **63**, 945–50.

James, J. E., Ziparo, V., Jeppsen, B., and Fischer, J. E. (1979) Hyper-ammonaemia, plasma amino acid imbalance and blood–brain amino acid transport: a unified theory of portal systemic encephalopathy. *Lancet*, **i**, 772–5.

James, W. P. T. (1982) Obesity, in *Nutrition and Health* Turner, M. R. (ed.), M.T.P. Press Ltd, ch. 9, 123–34.

Johnson-Sabine, E., Wakeling, A. (1983) Anorexia nervosa and related eating disorders. *Hospital Update*, **9**, 1341–53.

Kirby, D. F. and Craig, R. M. (1985) The value of intensive nutritional support in pancreatitis. *Journal of Parenteral and Enteral Nutrition*, **9**, 353–7.

Kopple, J. D., Massry, S. G., Olmer, M., and Heidland, A. (eds) (1983) Nutrition and metabolism in kidney disease. *Kidney*, **Supplement 16**.

Kromhout, D., Bosschieter, E. B., and Coulander, C. de L. (1985) The inverse reaction between fish consumption and 20 year mortality from coronary heart disease. *New England Journal of Medicine*, **312**, 1205–9.

Lucas, P. A., Meadows, J. H., Roberts, D. E., and Coles, G. A. (1986) The risks and benefits of a low protein/essential amino acid/keto acid diet. *Kidney International*, **29**, 95–1003.

Marmot, M. G., Rose, G., Shipley, M., and Hamilton, P. J. S. (1978) Employment grade and coronary heart disease in British civil servants. *Journal of Epidemiology and Community Health*, **32**, 244–61.

Meade, T. W. (1982) Diet, haemostatic function and ischaemic heart disease. In: Turner, M. R. (ed.) *Nutrition and Health* M.T.P. Press Ltd ch. 18, 231–41.

Miller, N. E. (1982) Biochemical and nutritional aspects of ischaemic heart disease: interactions between diet, lipoproteins and atherogenesis. In: Turner, M. R. (ed.) *Nutrition and Health* M.T.P. Press Ltd ch. 17, 219–30.

O'Morain, C., Segal, A. W., and Levi, A. J. (1984) Elemental diet as primary treatment of acute Crohn's disease. *British Journal of Medicine*, **288**, 1859–62.

Pafrey, P. S., Vandenburg, M. J., Wright, P., Holly, J. M. B., Goodwin, F. J., Evans, S. J. W., and Ledingham, J. M. (1981) Blood pressure and hormonal changes following alteration of dietary sodium and potassium in mild essential hypertension. *Lancet*, **i**, 59–63.

Palman, K. C. (1982) Cancer cachexia. *British Journal of Hospital Medicine*, **32**, 28–34.

Plant, M. A. (1982) Trends in alcohol consumption and alcohol-related problems in Britain. In: *Nutrition and Health*. Turner, M. R. (ed.) M.T.P. Press Ltd ch. 6, 71–86.

Simpson, H. R. C., Simpson, R. C., Lonsley, S., Carter, R. D., Geekie, M., Hockaday, T. D. R., and Mann, J. I. (1981) A high carbohydrate leguminous fibre diet improves all aspects of diabetic control. *Lancet*, **i**, 1–5.

Report of the Royal College of Physicians (1980) *Medical Aspects of Dietary Fibre*, Pitman Medical, Bath.

Thomson, A. D. and Mazumdar, S. K. (1982) The hazard to health from moderate drinking. *Nutrition and Health*. Turner, M. R. (ed.) M.T.P. Press Ltd ch. 7, 87–107.

Tunstall-Pedoe, H. (1982) Coronary heart disease prevention. In: Alwyn Smith (ed.) *Recent Advances in Community Medicine 2* Churchill Livingstone, Edinburgh. Ch. 8, 95–110.

8

DIET AND DISEASE

The food we eat can promote ill health in various ways. Inadequate nutrient intake will invariably lead to malnutrition and a poorly balanced diet is associated with a spectrum of disorders including intestinal and degenerative vascular disease. Food may be contaminated by micro-organisms and chemicals, and allergic or non-allergic reactions to specific food components may effect some patients. Malnutrition and methods of nutritional support, and the role of nutrition in genesis and management of disease have been discussed in earlier chapters. This chapter reviews the subject of food poisoning and food intolerance. It also includes a summary of therapeutic dietetics and outlines the principal diets in current use.

8.1 Food poisoning

Contamination of food with micro-organisms or their toxins is a frequent cause of illness, and agricultural chemicals or veterinary drugs may also enter human food. Radiation fall-out is a potential hazard emphasized by the recent Chernobyl disaster.

8.1.1 BACTERIAL CONTAMINATION OF FOOD

(a) Salmonella

(i) Salmonella infections There are more than 1400 different types of Salmonellae whose normal habitat is in the intestinal canal of a large

number of hosts. Those of animal origin cause the syndrome of gastroenteritis in their human victims. This illness is characterized by the simultaneous onset of vomiting and diarrhoea 12–48 hours after ingestion of contaminated food. The diarrhoea is secretory in type and dehydration is the main danger. The Salmonellae which predominantly reside in human intestines (Salmonella typhi and Salmonella paratyphi) produce an entirely different illness with fever and bacteraemia, in which diarrhoea is a later feature. The latter infections are usually found in underdeveloped countries and the tropics, but they are rare in Britain and will not be discussed further.

(ii) Food sources of Salmonellae Carcasses contaminated with Salmonellae pass from the abattoir to the meat factory. A small proportion of beef and pork sausages contains these organisms. Salmonellae are destroyed by cooking so that cooked or processed meats are safe provided that contamination does not subsequently occur from uncooked products. Poultry is a rich source of Salmonellae with a high rate of contamination, and these bacteria may also be found in duck eggs. Pasteurization is now compulsory for preserved egg products which are much used in confectionery and for synthetic creams. A breakdown in the pasteurization of milk has occasionally led to large outbreaks of salmonella gastroenteritis. Shellfish harvested from polluted waters are an obvious potential hazard, and rare outbreaks have been attributed to chocolate following contamination of the raw cocoa bean.

Episodes of salmonella infection are most commonly reported in the home or in restaurants due to inadequate food preparation. The incomplete thawing of frozen foods, especially chicken, allows the bacteria to survive cooking because of inadequate core temperatures. Storage of uncooked meats adjacent to cooked meats leads to contamination of the cooked product.

(b) Campylobacter infections

Campylobacter infections are usually acquired from poultry. The common modes of transmission involve inadequate cooking or contamination of cooked meat. Rarely, large milkborne outbreaks have followed a breakdown in the pasteurization process. After an incubation period of 2–5 days patients develop systemic symptoms of fever, myalgia and headache which are followed by abdominal pain and diarrhoea.

(c) Clostridium perfringens

This is primarily a soil organism which is widely distributed in nature. It is a common surface contaminant of raw meat, but is a strict anaerobe which only thrives in anaerobic conditions such as occur in cooked meats or stew. Most of the vegetative forms are killed by cooking but the organism forms spores which may survive for considerable periods at high temperatures. The presence of a few spores is of no consequence unless the meat is allowed to cool slowly through the temperature range of 50–20 °C. The spores will then germinate and the vegetative bacilli multiply rapidly. Following ingestion of the contaminated food these bacteria again form spores and in so doing produce an enterotoxin which is released when the organism is lyzed. The enterotoxin induces a secretory response, and so the patient typically develops abdominal pain and diarrhoea usually 12 hours after food ingestion.

(d) Staphylococci

This ubiquitous organism frequently colonizes the skin, and is a cause of skin sepsis which may lead to food contamination. At room temperature colonies grow rapidly and produce a heat-stable enterotoxin which resists subsequent cooking. Ingestion of contaminated food is followed by vomiting after 1–4 hours by a mechanism which involves the central nervous system. Confectionery, custards and creams, hams and pies are the foods which are most commonly affected.

(e) Bacillus cereus

This organism became notorious for infecting rice from Chinese restaurants. The rice is boiled in large batches during which spores are not killed. Subsequent storage of the rice for prolonged periods at room temperature facilitates spore germination and enterotoxin production. The vegetative bacilli and enterotoxins are not destroyed by rapid immersion in hot oil to produce fried rice. The unfortunate customer may develop one of two syndromes, early vomiting similar to that induced by staphylococcal toxin or later secretory diarrhoea as with Clostridial perfringens toxin.

(f) Vibrio parahaemolyticus

This is a food infection acquired from seafoods or shellfish, especially when they are eaten raw. Abdominal pain and diarrhoea are common features, but some patients also develop pyrexia, vomiting and headache.

(g) Miscellaneous bacteria

Many other bacteria may contaminate food, and they are listed in Table 8.1. Where sanitation and hygiene are poor, contamination with enterotoxigenic strains of Escherichia coli leads to a heat-stable toxin which induces diarrhoea. This is usually a mild illness which is described as traveller's diarrhoea. Conversely enteroinvasive Escherichia coli and Shigella species cause a more severe illness characterized by colonic mucosal invasion with bloody diarrhoea and fever. Vibrio cholera secretes a toxin that induces a severe secretory diarrhoea. These organisms usually cause disease in hot climates especially with impure water supplies. Uncooked vegetables or fruit washed in contaminated water are a potential source of infection.

Brucellosis is an infection of cows and goats which is transmitted by unpasteurized milk or cheese made from raw milk, and leads to a chronic pyrexial illness. In many parts of the world bovine tuberculosis is prevalent and the consumption of unpasteurized milk is a cause of gastrointestinal tuberculosis. Yersinia enterocolitica is an uncommon pathogen in Britain which has been isolated from meat, seafood and confectionery. It is a cause of gastroenteritis and ileocaecal inflammatory disease.

Botulism is a potentially lethal form of bacterial food poisoning which is now rare. Clostridium botulinum is a widespread saprophyte which produces heat-resistant spores. If these are not destroyed by adequate cooking vegetative forms grow in anaerobic conditions and produce a lethal toxin which blocks neuromuscular transmission. Weakness of cranial muscles may progress to respiratory paralysis. Home-canned meats are a potential hazard, and one of the reasons for the decline in this infection has been the introduction of cold storage for domestic meat preservation. The food industry uses nitrates to prevent anaerobic growth.

Table 8.1 Food and infection

Bacteria
  Bacillus cereus
  Brucella spp.
  Campylobacter spp.
  Clostridium botulinum
  Clostridium perfringens
  Escherichia coli
  Mycobacterium tuberculosis
  Salmonella spp.
  Shigella spp.
  Staphylococci
  Vibrio parahaemolyticus
  Vibrio cholera
  Yersinia
Protozoa
  Entamoeba histolytica
  Giardia lamblia
Viruses
  Hepatitis A
  Norwalk agent
  Polio virus
  Rota virus
Helminths
  Clonorchis spp.
  Diphyllobothrium latum
  Fasciola hepatica
  Taenia saginata
  Taenia solium
  Trichinella spp.

8.1.2 VIRAL AND PROTOZOAL INFECTIONS

(a) Viral infections

The Rota and Norwalk viruses are common causes of gastroenteritis which may be transmitted by food handlers, dirty utensils or contaminated water. Whereas bacteria usually induce a toxin-mediated secretory diarrhoea, viruses frequently damage the small intestinal mucosa and cause temporary malabsorption. The Rota virus in particular can lead to lactose malabsorption in children. Typically diarrhoea recurs when milk is reintroduced and the diagnosis is supported by testing for reducing substances in the stool. The problem is remedied by the temporary use of low lactose milk substitutes such as Pregestemil. Some paediatricians use this routinely following such infections until the stools become normal when milk is gradually reintroduced.

The hepatitis A virus is also transmitted by the faecal oral route. The ingestion of contaminated water or seafood obtained in the vicinity of sewage effluent can lead to viral hepatitis after 2–6 weeks. The majority of such infections are subclinical. Icteric or rarely fulminant hepatitis may ensue but this infection does not lead to chronic liver disease.

(b) Protozoa

Giardia lamblia is a protozoan which contaminates food and water supplies. It is not uncommon in Britain but it is particularly prevalent in parts of the world where human sewage is spread on the land. Infection may be asymptomatic, some patients suffer from nausea, abdominal pain and diarrhoea, and others develop steatorrhoea. The condition may be confirmed by finding cysts in the stool or trophozoites in duodenal aspirates.

Entamoeba histolytica is transmitted in a similar fashion to Giardia, and usually only occurs in British patients after a visit to the tropics. The organism attacks the colon to produce a syndrome of bloody diarrhoea which can be mistaken for ulcerative colitis if stool microscopy is omitted. Occasionally it is carried in the portal venous blood to form a hepatic abscess. Both of these protozoal infections respond to Metronidazole.

8.1.3 WORM INFESTATIONS

Three categories of worm infestation are recognized: nematodes (round worms), cestodes (tape worms) and trematodes (flukes).

(a) Nematode infections

Examples of nematode infections include Ascaris lumbricoides, species of Enterobiasis, and Trichuris trichuria in which eggs are ingested following the faecal contamination of food. Adult worms can be identified in the stool.

(b) Cestode infections

Cestodes are acquired when the larval form is ingested, usually in undercooked beef (Taenia saginata) or pork (Taenia solium). The cysticercus is liberated in the small intestine, the head attaches itself to the gut wall and the adult develops by proliferating thousands of segments. Eggs are passed in the faeces and if ingested by the respective animal host the liberated embryo enters the bloodstream and settles in the tissues where it develops into cysticerci.

Most patients are symptomless but become aware of infection when segments are observed in the stool. However the larval phase of Taenia solium can exist in human tissue, a condition called cysticercosis. Cysticercosis develops when eggs are transmitted from the anus to the mouth or by the liberation of many eggs in the intestine following the disintegration of the tapeworm with treatment.

The ingestion of uncooked fish can cause infestation with Diphyllobothrium latum. This may cause a megaloblastic anaemia by impairing the absorption of Vitamin B12.

(c) Trematode infestations

Schistosomiasis is the most common example of trematode infestation but this is not a foodborne disease. The liver fluke Fasciola hepatica is common in sheep, and has been reported in humans who acquired it by eating contaminated watercress.

8.1.4 FOOD TOXINS

(a) Fungal toxins

Many species of mushrooms are toxic and contain active ingredients which irritate the alimentary tract, stimulate the central nervous system, or damage the kidneys and liver. Symptoms of nausea, vomiting and diarrhoea usually begin shortly after ingestion. Most serious and fatal intoxications are caused by Amanita phalloides which may lead to renal, hepatic and intestinal failure through cyclic peptides which block ribonucleic acid synthesis. Poisoning is usually accidental when such mushrooms are mistaken for edible varieties. However some genera such as Canocybe produce pleasant hallucinations and a state of euphoria, and are sometimes used for self-intoxication.

Claviceps species may contaminate grain in damp environments, and they can produce ergot alkaloids which in the past led to outbreaks of disease characterized by severe burning pains in the limbs with subsequent gangrene, known as St. Anthony's fire. Nuts and grain stored in humid conditions may become contaminated by Aspergillus flavus which produces aflotoxin. Aflotoxins cause hepatic damage and ultimately hepatic carcinoma in the laboratory animal, so there has been speculation about their importance in areas where this tumour is common. Recently it has been suggested that the ingestion of small amounts of aflotoxin may be one reason why some malnourished patients develop the features of kwashiorkor rather than marasmus.

(b) Toxins from seafood

Bacterial contamination of tuna or mackerel may lead to the formation of histamine from the histidine which is liberated by damaged muscle. This causes headaches, flushing and diarrhoea shortly after ingestion and these symptoms are not prevented by cooking. Occasionally mussels may contain saxitoxin which causes weakness, paraesthesia, ataxia and vomiting within 30 minutes of ingestion, with a risk of death from respiratory paralysis. Some neurotoxins which induce weakness and paraesthesia have been associated with the ingestion of many species of fish in the Pacific Ocean and Caribbean Sea; these fish have usually been feeding on coral reefs.

(c) Miscellaneous food toxins

Potatoes contain small amounts of solanine which is concentrated in the skin, eyes and sprouts. This chemical is water soluble so that negligible amounts are ingested from potatoes which have been peeled and boiled. However larger concentrations of solanine are formed in and beneath the skin when potatoes are exposed to light during growth or storage. If such potatoes are baked in their skins serious solanine poisoning may ensue. Symptoms include headaches, fever, vomiting, abdominal pain and diarrhoea. Recovery usually occurs over a few days. The suggested association of solanine ingestion with neural tube defects in utero has yet to be established.

Cabbage and other members of the Brassica genus contain thiocyanates and glucosinolates which respectively inhibit iodine concentration and thyroxine synthesis by the thyroid gland. There is no evidence that this vegetable is harmful when ingested in normal amounts, rather it is a valuable nutrient source as discussed in Chapter 3. Sanguinarine is derived from a poppy weed which can contaminate crops of mustard seed and groundnuts that are grown for their oil. It inhibits the oxidation of pyruvate and may lead to cardiomyopathy. Affected individuals develop oedema.

8.1.5 RADIOACTIVE FALL-OUT

Atmospheric nuclear explosions between 1945 and 1963 and accidents at nuclear power stations like those at Windscale in 1957 and Chernobyl in 1986 have liberated large amounts of radioactive dust into the atmosphere. This eventually settles on the earth's surface over distances of many thousands of miles. Radioactive fall-out contaminates crops and pasture land and thus animals. Food of animal origin is potentially more hazardous because of the concentration of radioactivity in milk and meat.

The most important radio-isotopes in this context are Iodine 131, Strontium 90, and Caesium 137 with respective half lives of 8 days, 28 and 30 years. Iodide administration may block radioactive uptake by the thyroid gland. Strontium is particularly dangerous because it has a long half life, it is secreted in milk, and it is stored in bone close to the marrow. Increasing dietary calcium may reduce strontium uptake because of a shared transport mechanism.

8.1.6 MISCELLANEOUS CONTAMINANTS

Modern agricultural methods involve the use of many chemicals. Pesticides such as DDT and Dieldrin persist in agricultural products and may be ingested with food. The finding of significant amounts of these substances in human fat led to a restriction of their use for livestock and food crops. The use of fungicides such as alkyl mercury on seed grain has caused human poisoning when such grain has been used in baking or for chicken feed.

The misuse of antibiotics in animal husbandry to promote growth is now illegal. Previously it was responsible for emerging bacterial resistance to a wide range of antibiotics, resistance which can be passed to human pathogens. The inadvertent consumption of antibiotics may still occur through veterinary practice, for example Penicillin used to treat infection in cattle may contaminate milk and thus lead to illness in patients with a previous history of Penicillin sensitivity. Diethylstilboestrol is no longer permitted for the enhancement of animal growth after the demonstration that oestrogens can be transferred to humans via meat.

Many chemicals are added to preserve or enhance the flavour or colour of food, and they are discussed in Chapter 3. All have been extensively tested but some such as monosodium glutamate and tartrazine may cause illness, a subject which is discussed later in this chapter.

8.1.7 THE PREVENTION OF FOOD POISONING

The quality and safety of food sold for human consumption has been the subject of extensive legislation in many countries. This is primarily concerned with the prevention of contamination by harmful micro-organisms or chemicals. More recent developments include an obligation to list the ingredients, including additives, of processed food and the need to indicate the date by which pre-packed food should be sold or consumed.

Conditions in the shop will often determine the quality of food reaching the customer. The effect of temperature can be critical, as a warm environment will facilitate rapid multiplication of a few remaining Clostridia or Salmonellae in meat products or Staphylococci in cream. Inappropriate storage where cooked meats are placed alongside uncooked meat or poultry is very dangerous. Infection may also be spread by flies, vermin or even food handlers. In some developed countries legislation exists to ensure that people who develop gastroenteritis are not allowed to return to work in the food industry until adequate bacteriological examination has established clearance of the offending organism.

Standards of hygiene and the principles of cooking, cooling and storing food are increasingly taught to people entering the catering industry. In some countries legislation permits the closure of restaurants where the kitchens do not measure up to modern requirements.

8.2 Food intolerance

Adverse reactions to food may occur because it contains toxins, some of which have been discussed previously. Alternatively intolerance to dietary components which are generally non-toxic may develop in some patients. Food intolerance is sometimes psychogenic. Organic causes involve allergic and non-allergic mechanisms. This represents a controversial area of clinical practice in which the placebo effect and observer bias have sometimes led to unsubstantiated claims.

8.2.1 FOOD ALLERGY

(a) Spectrum of disease

Food allergy most commonly affects young children, and its role in the pathogenesis of many diseases has now been confirmed. Some of these conditions are listed in Table 8.2. Gluten enteropathy (coeliac disease) is entirely related to the dietary ingestion of gluten, and colitis in young children may be caused by milk. Allergy to food is but one of several factors which may trigger angio-oedema, urticaria, rhinorrhoea and asthma.

In addition to these specific syndromes food allergy may be responsible for a variety of symptoms. They include perioral itching,

Table 8.2 Conditions associated with food allergy

General
    Anaphylaxis
    Angio-oedema
Gastrointestinal
    Gluten enteropathy
    Colitis (in infants)
Respiratory
    Rhinitis
    Asthma
Dermatological
    Urticaria
    Eczema
    Dermatitis herpetiformis

rhinorrhoea, vomiting, abdominal pain, diarrhoea and steatorrhoea. The latter may be a feature of temporary intolerance, frequently to cow's milk which occurs in children after viral gastroenteritis. Lip swelling, rhinorrhoea and vomiting occur within a few minutes of food ingestion, asthma and urticaria within an hour, and diarrhoea develops later. Such features usually settle within one day. Gluten enteropathy and eczema develop and progress over prolonged periods.

(b) Foods most commonly incriminated

The foods most commonly responsible for allergic symptoms are cow's milk, eggs, nuts, shellfish, and wheat. Other items such as chocolate, pork, chicken and artificial colourings are sometimes incriminated.

(c) The diagnosis of food allergy

Establishing a diagnosis of food allergy, like food hypersensitivity, is dependent upon the clinical history. Laboratory tests including skin tests and radio–allergosorbent (RAST) tests are unreliable because of false negatives and false positives.

In the classical case of anaphylaxis following shellfish ingestion the symptoms are dramatic and immediate and the diagnosis is obvious. When the diagnosis is uncertain dietary cards may be of value. The patient keeps an accurate record of all foods and drinks and a second record of the time, nature and duration of symptoms. Analysis of the food record may incriminate one or more items. Subsequently the patient is asked to continue with the records but to omit the suspect foods from the diet. Such an approach is unsuccessful in patients with frequent symptoms who are allergic or intolerant of several food items. Under these circumstances it is necessary to use an elimination diet.

An example of an elimination diet is given in Table 8.3. The patient remains on the basic diet until symptoms have settled for up to two weeks. Thereafter one new food item is introduced every three days, with small quantities on the first day and normal servings on subsequent days. If no reactions are experienced on three consecutive days the item is allowed freely in the diet thereafter. Conversely if any reactions occur no more of the food is taken and the patient is asked to

Table 8.3   The basic elimination diet

Lamb:	Fresh or pure frozen lamb, e.g. lamb chops, minced lamb, stewing lamb
Turkey:	Fresh or pure frozen turkey. Avoid turkey roll and turkey roast – they contain other foods
Vegetables:	Only the following six vegetables are allowed: carrot, turnip, cauliflower, cabbage, celery, brussels sprouts
Potato:	Boiled, baked, roast or fried in permitted oils
Rice:	Long grain, short grain, brown and white rice. Also ground rice and rice flour. Rice cakes (available from health food shops). Rice Krispies
Permitted flours:	Rice flour, potato flour, sago flour, and buckwheat
Fruit:	Pears and pineapple, fresh or tinned
Drinks:	Weak tea, water. Pure pineapple juice. '7 UP' lemonade
Miscellaneous:	Tomor margarine, Granose margarine. Sugar, honey, syrup, treacle. Olive oil, sunflower oil. Sea salt, fresh ground pepper, pure herbs

wait until the symptoms settle before introducing another food. During the introduction period a diary of foods introduced and reactions or symptoms are noted and at the end the patient submits a summary sheet as shown in Table 8.4.

The use of an elimination diet has many pitfalls. Successful application requires an intelligent and conscientious patient, and the restrictive diet is inconvenient and disruptive of family routine over a prolonged period. It may encourage unhealthy introspection, patients frequently lose weight, and interpretation can be confused by neurotic traits. Consequently the desirability of establishing the diagnosis by subjecting food items, suspected on the basis of clinical history, dietary cards or elimination diets, to provocation merits emphasis. Ideally this should be done on more than one occasion with the study

Table 8.4   Elimination diet summary sheet

Name..

Date of birth ....

Date basic elimination diet started..

Foods introduced	Date	Reaction yes/no type
Beef		
Chicken		
Pork		
Bacon/ham		
Soya milk		
Apple		
Banana		
Orange		
Tomato		
Corn		
Oats		
Onion		
Baked beans		
Peas		
Fish		
Wheat		
Yeast		
Eggs		
Cow's milk		
Chocolate		
Peanuts		

and control food delivered through naso-gastric tubes. However, many patients who have successfully and reasonably incriminated one or two food items prefer simply to omit these from their diet and are not prepared to undergo such laborious testing. Furthermore these challenges should not be given to patients who suffer from symptoms which are potentially dangerous such as anaphylaxis or angioneurotic reactions. Nevertheless care must be taken to ensure that neurotic patients do not eat restricted and nutritionally unsatisfactory diets on the basis of imagined and non-existent allergies.

(d) The treatment of food allergy

Foods which provoke severe symptoms should be omitted. This is readily achieved with items such as shellfish which are eaten infrequently. It is more difficult with common foods like cow's milk and eggs. Some patients may be able to tolerate goat's milk, others may find soya milk preferable. Occasionally denaturing the proteins by boiling milk or boiling eggs for 10 minutes rather than the customary 3–4 minutes prevents reactions. Hyposensitization is of no value. The prophylactic administration of oral chromoglycate has been used in patients who have many allergies so that avoidance of all offending food items is impractical. The ingestion of the contents of 2–4 capsules dissolved in warm water 30 minutes before eating has been recommended, but it is not always successful. The development of severe reactions sush as asthma or angioneurotic oedema or anaphylaxis may require the use of corticosteroids, Salbutamol or even adrenaline.

8.2.2 FOOD HYPERSENSITIVITY

Some patients are intolerant of specific foods because of non-immunogenic mechanisms which are often poorly defined. The following are examples of food intolerance due to food hyper-sensitivity.

- Hypersensitivity to coffee may provoke cardiac irregularity and cause the patient to complain of palpitations. The use of decaffeinated coffee and the avoidance of strong tea and caffeine-containing soft drinks is all that is required.
- The vasomotor activity of amines appears to provoke vascular headaches similar to migraine in susceptible subjects who need to avoid foods rich in tyramine such as cheese
- Monosodium glutamate, a flavouring enhancer which is widely used by the food industry in savoury foods, leads to transient symptoms in a minority of consumers who describe numbness, weakness, burning sensations and palpitations

- Food colouring such as tartrazine can provoke urticaria in susceptible patients

Some forms of food intolerance are controversial. For example there is evidence that food additives such as tartrazine provoke hyperactivity in some children. Although many authorities dispute the concept of food intolerance in the pathogenesis of hyperactivity, a proportion of affected children appear to benefit from additive-free diets. Also a proportion of patients with the irritable bowel syndrome claim that their symptoms are provoked or aggravated by food items such as wheat, coffee, dairy produce or citrus fruits. Sometimes it is necessary to resort to diary cards or elimination diets to substantiate these claims. It has been observed that such patients who commence the elimination diet can initially suffer an exacerbation of symptoms and may not feel well until after the first week.

Even more caution is required before accepting food intolerance as the explanation for numerous symptoms including tiredness, oedema, arthralgia, bruising, dizziness and palpitations. Such patients are usually depressed and are seeking a more acceptable explanation for psychiatric disease. If these patients are investigated by the previously described techniques it is essential that any apparent food intolerance is formally substantiated. Failure to do so will increase the patient's problems by restricting their diet and distracting attention from the main reason for their illness.

8.2.3 ENZYME DEFICIENCIES

(a) Lactase deficiency

Different types of lactase deficiency are recognized. Congenital isolated deficiency is extremely rare. Acquired post-weaning lactase deficiency affects older children and adults, and is uncommon in Western Europe. Some patients have sub-clinical hypolactasia and only develop symptoms after gastric surgery. Reversible lactase deficiency may complicate viral gastroenteritis. Viruses can damage the intestinal mucosa and lead to increased cell turnover, lactase is present in mature enterocytes.

Lactase deficiency allows lactose to enter the large intestine where it is metabolized by colonic bacteria to hydrogen, carbon dioxide and organic acids. The latter induce an osmotic diarrhoea. Affected

patients also complain of adominal pain and distension, excess flatus
and borborygmus. Lactose intolerance is confirmed by lactose challenge. Lactase deficiency can then be established by measuring blood
glucose, breath hydrogen and stool pH (reducing substances are
identified by Clinitest). Lactase can be measured in jejunal biopsies,
but the mucosa must be histologically normal before the result can be
interpreted.

(b) Glucose 6-phosphate dehydrogenase deficiency

This genotype is found in up to 30% of some Mediterranean
populations and 10% of American negroes. The enzyme promotes the
stability of the red cell membrane, and haemolytic anaemia develops
when affected individuals are treated with oxidant drugs such as
sulphonamides and some anti-malarials. The ingestion of broad beans
can produce the same effect and continued ingestion will cause severe
anaemia described in the Mediterranean countries as favism.

8.3 Therapeutic dietetics

There is accumulating evidence that changes in the national diet may
significantly reduce the incidence of many diseases including diabetes,
hypertension, ischaemic heart disease and diverticular disease. This
subject is discussed in Chapter 7. There is a revival of interest in the use
of therapeutic diets as one aspect of the treatment of disease. This
subject is briefly reviewed, but for more detailed discussion the reader
is referred to standard textbooks of dietetics.

The diets in common use are listed in Table 8.5. Each diet should
provide all required essential nutrients in appropriate proportions in
relation to the disease for which is it prescribed. In particular it must be
suitable for the patient with respect to cost, personal preference and
any religious obligation. Frequently this calls for ingenuity on the part
of the dietitian who must have a knowledge of the nutritional
implications of disease, the nutritional requirements of the patient,
and the nutrient content of food. Especially important is the ability to
communicate in a practical, persuasive and interesting way. Rigid
dietary impositions and reduced palatability lead to difficulties of
interpretation and compliance, particularly as these restrictions can
affect the dietary habits of the entire family. Frequent advice and
encouragement is needed by a dietitian who is prepared to construct a

Table 8.5 Examples of therapeutic diets and their applications

Diet	Clinical indication
Energy reduced	Obesity. Diabetes in overweight patients
Energy increased	Malnutrition. Trauma. Sepsis
High protein	Nephrosis. Protein losing enteropathy
High fibre	Constipation. Diverticular disease
Fluid diets	Fractured jaw. Dysphagia due to oesophageal stricture
Diabetic diets	Insulin dependent and maturity onset diabetes
Low animal fat	Hypercholesterolaemia
Low protein	Uraemia. Portal systemic encephalopathy
Low sodium	Oedema of cardiac, renal or hepatic origin
Low potassium	Renal failure
Elimination diet	Food intolerance or allergy
Additive free diet	Urticaria. Hyperactivity
Wheat free	Wheat intolerance
Gluten free	Gluten enteropathy Dermatitis herpetiformis
Milk free	Milk allergy. Lactase deficiency
Ketogenic diet	Resistant myoclonic epilepsy

diet for the individual patient, based on likes and dislikes, by reference to food tables to provide a palatable and varied menu.

8.3.1 LOW ENERGY DIETS

Energy-reduced diets for the management of obesity usually contain 1000 kcal (4.2 MJ) less than the estimated daily requirements. Thus adult females are advised to eat 1000 kcal (4.2 MJ) per day, and males are allowed 1500 kcal (6.3 MJ). Foods can conveniently be considered in three categories as illustrated in Table 8.6, those which should be avoided, those which are unrestricted, and those which are available in limited amounts.

(a) Foods which should be avoided

Energy-dense foods are not allowed. These include sugary foods such as sweets, ice cream and dried fruits, starchy foods such as cakes and

Table 8.6 Low energy diet: categories of foods

Foods to avoid

Sugary food	Sugar, honey, jam, marmalade, syrup, chocolate, sweets, packet desserts, tinned fruit, ice cream, fruit yoghurt, dried fruits
Starchy food	Cakes, biscuits, pastry, batter, custard, semolina, sago, tapioca, oatmeal
Fatty foods	Fatty meat e.g. streaky bacon, sausage rolls, pies and rissoles, chips, crisps, roast potatoes, nuts, cream, mayonnaise, all fried foods

Foods which are unlimited

Green vegetables	Cabbage, cauliflower, French and runner beans, broccoli, spinach, brussels sprouts, leeks, asparagus
Salad vegetables	Lettuce, tomato, cucumber, spring onions, celery, peppers
Root vegetables	Carrots, onions, swede, turnip
Miscellaneous vegetables	Marrow, aubergines, courgettes, mushrooms
Beverages	Bovril, marmite, tea, coffee, tomato juice, grapefruit juice (unsweetened), low calorie squashes
Condiments	Salt, pepper, mustard, vinegar, Worcester sauce, curry powder, herbs

Foods which are rationed

Meat	Poultry, game, mince, beef, liver, lamb, pork
Fish	Cod, lemon sole, whiting, herring, kipper, mackerel, pilchards
Miscellaneous	Bread, peas, parsnips, fruit, potatoes, rice

---

pastries, fatty foods like chips, and cream as well as beverages like beer and milk drinks. Patients who require sweet foods may use non-calorific artifical sweeteners such as saccharin. Artificial sweeteners are discussed in Section 8.3.6.

(b) Foods which are unrestricted

There is no limit to the consumption of green vegetables such as cabbage, sprouts, runner beans or broccoli, salad vegetables like lettuce, tomatoes, and cucumber and root vegetables including carrots, onions, swede and turnip. Patients are also allowed free access to selected beverages such as meat and yeast extracts, tea or coffee, and sugar-free carbonated drinks and lemonade are also allowed.

(c) Foods which are rationed

Meat, poultry, fish, cheese, eggs, milk and butter or margarine are chosen from a daily allowance the amount of which will be determined by the desired energy restriction.

(d) The well-balanced low energy diet

The patient is encouraged to eat three meals a day, not to eat between meals, and to choose from each of the main categories of food while avoiding the energy-dense foods listed in Table 8.6. A daily amount of restricted foods is defined: the amount is determined by the energy restriction, and the relative proportions of the individual items by the patient's preferences. A sample 1000 kcal (4.2 MJ) diet is illustrated in Table 8.7. Many patients will not need such detailed dietary instruction. For them the avoidance of energy-dense foods and eating between meals is sufficient to promote desired weight loss.

8.3.2 HIGH ENERGY DIETS

The provision of large energy-dense meals for the malnourished, ill or convalescent patient is frequently impractical because of anorexia or intestinal intolerance. The majority of patients in this category require skilful dietetic and nursing management to ensure an adequate nutrient intake. Many patients respond best to moderate-sized meals with additional snacks of milk drinks or sandwiches mid morning, mid afternoon and at bedtime. Energy consumption can also be increased by the addition of milk or cream to soups or sauces, butter or margarine to potatoes, vegetables and scrambled eggs, sugar or glucose to drinks, puddings, and fruit.

8.3.3 HIGH PROTEIN DIETS

Patients who require high protein diets are encouraged to drink 600–800 ml of milk a day which can be flavoured by coffee, ovaltine,

Table 8.7 Energy-reduced diet (1000 kcal: 4.2 MJ)

A sample menu

Breakfast	½ grapefruit or 100 ml unsweetened fruit juice 20 g of high fibre breakfast cereal or 120 g of porridge with milk from allowance 1 thin slice of wholemeal bread with butter or margarine from allowance
Mid morning	Coffee or tea with milk from allowance
Lunch	Clear soup 30 g cheese or 1 egg 2 thin slices of wholemeal bread with butter from allowance 1 piece or serving of fruit
Mid afternoon	Tea or coffee with milk from allowance
Dinner	100 ml of tomato or unsweetened fruit juice 60 g lean meat or chicken or 90 g white fish 2 boiled potatoes Salad or boiled vegetables 2 wafers or crispbread with margarine or butter from allowance 1 serving of fruit Coffee with milk from allowance
Evening	Tea or coffee with milk from allowance or another permitted beverage
Daily allowance	300 ml skimmed milk 15 g butter or margarine

chocolate or milk shake syrup. Some patients may prefer to substitute a carton of yogurt for 150 ml of milk. Cooked breakfasts should be provided with bacon and egg or fish, as well as generous helpings of meat, fish and cheese with the main meals. Build-Up, Complan or 'egg flip' are useful high protein drinks which can be taken between meals. Such diets must be accompanied by an increase in the energy intake.

Common indications for high protein diets include the nephrotic syndrome and malnutrition associated with alcohol addiction. These patients are often hypoalbuminaemic and oedematous and require salt restriction. Under these circumstances highly salted protein sources should be avoided including ham, bacon, sausages, smoked fish and cheese, and unsalted butter should be used.

8.3.4 HIGH FIBRE DIETS

Patients are advised to eat high fibre cereals in the form of wholemeal bread and bran-enriched bread, and wholegrain breakfast cereals including All-Bran, Weetabix and muesli. Wholegrain or bran biscuits such as digestive, Ryvita and oatcakes replace more refined products, and wholemeal flour, pasta and brown rice are used.

All kinds of fruit should be eaten especially dried fruit such as prunes and pears and apples including the skins. Patients are encouraged to take liberal helpings of vegetables and potatoes, when baked, should be eaten with their skins. Unprocessed bran can be added to breakfast cereals or soups to give more fibre. Patients vary in their requirement and tolerance, so whereas two heaped table-spoonsful is the usual recommendation a smaller quantity is introduced first and increased gradually to avoid the abdominal discomfort and excessive flatulence experienced by patients who are accustomed to low dietary fibre.

8.3.5 FLUID DIETS

Some patients manage to take normal food after it has been liquidized, others with more advanced dysphagia or fractured jaws need liquid diets. Breakfast may consist of fruit juice, thin strained porridge with milk, egg in milk or Complan or Build-Up. The two main meals include strained soup, thin milk pudding, ice cream or yogurt. Milk shakes, hot chocolate or high protein drinks are used to supplement the main meals or as an additional snack. Alternatively whole protein polymeric liquid feeds may be preferred, flavoured according to the patient's preference. Such diets lack bulk and can cause colonic dysfunction. Some polymeric diets are now available with fibre supplements and these may prove useful. These preparations are discussed in Chapter 5. Liquid diets for patients whose jaws have been wired for the management of obesity must be selected to avoid the provision of excess energy.

8.3.6 DIABETIC DIETS

(a) Non-insulin dependent diabetes

Many elderly non-insulin dependent diabetics can be managed effectively by the avoidance of sugar, sweets and other sources of energy-dense highly refined carbohydrate. They are subsequently able to tolerate more carbohydrate provided it is of an unrefined type.

Patients must be instructed not only to avoid white and brown sugar but also jam, honey, chocolate spread and sweet cakes, pastries and buns. Sugar-coated breakfast cereals, tinned fruits, soft drinks and sweet sherry and wine are also to be avoided. When possible the patient should be encouraged to adapt to non-sweetened foods and drinks. Those who retain a preference for sweet foods can use artificial sweetener.

Natural calorific sweeteners include fructose which is almost twice as sweet as glucose, and lactose and sorbitol which are less sweet. Sorbitol may induce diarrhoea, and xylitol is an alternative currently under investigation. Aspartane (Canderel, Nutra-Sweet) is up to 200 times sweeter than glucose with a more persistent taste. It is unstable in aqueous solution and at high temperature, and because one of the constituents is phenylalanine it should not be used in patients with phenylketonuria. These preparations are best avoided by patients who are overweight. They should use the synthetic non-calorific sweetener saccharin (Hermesetas, Saxin or Sweetex). The granulated sweeteners (Sucron, Sweet and Low) should not be used by diabetics.

A significant number of non-insulin dependent diabetics are obese. Weight loss is difficult to achieve in this group but it leads to improved glucose tolerance. Such patients should be managed by energy-reduced diets which are discussed in Section 8.3.1.

(b) Insulin dependent diabetes

The diet and management of insulin dependent diabetes has until recently been influenced by two misconceptions. Firstly the belief that the disease simply reflects glucose intolerance led to the restriction of carbohydrate and the provision of more energy from fat, a policy which may have enhanced atherogenesis. Secondly no attention was paid to the different glycaemic response to refined and unrefined carbohydrate. Current dietary advice emphasises the increased

provision of carbohydrate energy and the use of unrefined carbohydrate sources. The total energy provision will be normal, increased
or decreased depending upon the patient's weight. The distribution of
the energy in meals and snacks throughout the day depends upon the
type of insulin regime the patient requires (see Table 7.2). This is
discussed more fully in Chapter 7.

The diet is regulated using a system of exchanges. Each exchange is
defined as 10 g of carbohydrate. Every patient receives a complete list
of foods with a convenient measure that corresponds to one exchange.
A sample list is shown in Table 8.8. The total number of exchanges
allowed each day is governed by the total energy requirement bearing
in mind that 70% of this should be provided as carbohydrate. The
number of exchanges in each meal will depend on the insulin regime.
Patients are taught to select carbohydrate food with care and to
include wholemeal cereals, vegetables, fruit and skimmed milk as the
main sources. Such items as white bread, plain biscuits, nuts, cream

Table 8.8 Convenient measures of food which contain one 10 g
exchange of carbohydrate

Food	Measure
Bread	1 small slice, ½ large slice
Digestive biscuit	1 large, 2 small
Cream crackers	2
Oatcakes	1 large, 1½ small
Bran flakes	5 tablespoons
Porridge	7 tablespoons
Muesli (unsweetened)	2 tablespoons
Spaghetti	40 g
Macaroni	40 g
Cooked rice	2 tablespoons
Chips	5
Boiled potato	1 small
Baked beans	5 tablespoons
Apple	1 small
Orange	1 medium
Milk	1 glass (200 ml)
Milk pudding	3 tablespoons
Ice cream	1 scoop

soups, black puddings, sausages and pies, should only be selected occasionally. Sweets, sweet cordials, tinned fruit and sugar-coated breakfast cereals must be avoided. An example of a diabetic diet is given in Table 8.9.

Table 8.9 A sample menu for insulin dependent diabetics: amount of food determined by energy allowance

Breakfast
    Wholegrain cereal or porridge
    Fish or grilled bacon
    Wholemeal toast
    Tea or coffee with milk from allowance

Mid morning
    Digestive or high fibre biscuit
    Tea or coffee with milk from allowance

Main meal
    Clear soup
    Meat or fish
    Potatoes
    Vegetables
    Fruit
    Biscuits and cheese

Mid afternoon
    Digestive or high fibre biscuit
    Tea or coffee with milk from allowance

Main meal
    Meat or fish
    Vegetables or salad
    Potatoes
    Fruit
    Tea or coffee with milk from allowance

Supper
    Cheese or meat sandwich or biscuit
    Tea or coffee or milk from allowance

8.3.7 LOW ANIMAL FAT DIET

Patients who require low animal fat diets should restrict their total fat consumption to less than 30% of their energy needs and ideally two thirds of this fat intake should be in the form of polyunsaturates. This can be achieved by avoiding foods which are rich in saturated fats and limiting the intake of other fat-containing items.

(a) Foods to be avoided

This list includes fatty meats such as pâté, sausages, pies, luncheon meat, tongue, duck, and goose, and fatty fish such as mackerel and sardines in oil. All fried meats and fish are not permitted, wholemilk, fried eggs and all hard and cream cheese, butter, cream and suet are not allowed. Potatoes should not be eaten fried, roasted or chipped; pastries, puddings and cakes made with wholemilk, cream and eggs are also avoided. Other forbidden foods include coconut, peanut butter, lemon curd, chocolate and fudge.

(b) Foods which can be eaten in moderation

Patients may eat moderate amounts of lean meat, Edam cheese and margarine rich in polyunsaturates. They are allowed three whole eggs per week. The occasional consumption of shellfish, chips fried in polyunsaturated oil, cakes, pastries and biscuits made from polyunsaturated margarine is allowed.

(c) Unrestricted foods

Patients may choose freely from a list of items including poultry, white fish, egg whites, cottage cheese, skimmed milk, wholemeal cereals, fruit and vegetables except avocados. Wholemeal bread, meringues, plain biscuits, and fatless sponge require no restriction. The same applies to jams, honey and boiled sweets.

Patients should be given such lists of foods and advised to scrutinize carefully the contents of convenience foods. The avoidance of some food categories and the restriction of food intake from other groups may reduce blood cholesterol values, but some patients require more detailed and stringent dietary advice.

8.3.8 PROTEIN RESTRICTION

(a) Very low protein diets

Very low protein diets which provide approximately 20 g of protein, originally introduced by Giovannetti, are no longer in common use due to the wide availability of renal dialysis, although some patients with portal systemic encephalopathy may require this type of diet which involves severe restriction of all foods which contain protein. For example they may have an allowance of 200 ml of milk, 40 g of meat, and 180 g of potatoes. They must eat low protein bread, very low protein vegetables and fruit such as tomatoes, carrots, green beans, pears, apples, and grapefruit. Additional sources of non-protein energy are needed: these include Hycal, Caloreen and Maxijual. Double cream was traditionally used to increase the energy content but the need to avoid the consumption of excessive saturated fats should be considered. Furthermore fruits and potatoes contain significant amounts of potassium and may require substitution in renal patients by fruit squashes and rice.

(b) Low protein diets

The majority of patients with chronic renal failure of moderate severity of portal systemic encephalopathy are managed with a 40 g protein diet. Such a diet is based upon a daily allowance of protein foods with emphasis on high class proteins, such as the example shown in Table 8.10. A variety of cakes and biscuits containing 2 g of protein can be substituted for one slice of bread. Suitable low protein vegetables include green beans, beetroot, cabbage, carrots, mushrooms, tomatoes and turnip. Most fruits can be eaten. The precise

Table 8.10 Protein restriction: an example of some allowances for a 40 g diet

Food	Allowance	Protein (g)
Milk	300 ml	9
Meat	90 g	21
Potato	180 g	3
Bread	90 g	7.5

structure of the diet will depend on the patient's preferences and to assist compliance patients are given a list of free and forbidden foods as illustrated in Table 8.11.

More liberal protein allowances of 60 g a day are occasionally used to prevent patients with chronic liver disease developing portal system encephalopathy by over-indulging in heavy protein meals. In future these diets may have a role in retarding the progression of chronic renal failure. Also under evaluation is the use of essential amino acid supplements or their keto acid analogues in order to expand the range of protein sources to include vegetable proteins. Indeed there is evidence that patients with portal systemic encephalopathy improve when their diet is changed from animal to vegetable protein sources.

Table 8.11 Foods list for patients on protein-restricted diets

Free foods

Sugars	Sugar, glucose Jam, marmalade, honey, syrup Boiled sweets, barley sugars, peppermints, all fruit sweets and ice lollies
Cereals	Cornflour, custard powder, sago, tapioca
Fats	Butter, margarine, lard, cooking fat, oil, cream
Vegetables	All vegetables *except* peas, beans, lentils
Beverages	Tea, coffee, instant coffee, Coffeemate, fruit juice, squash, lemonade, cordials
Fruit	Fresh, stewed and canned
Miscellaneous	Pepper, mustard, vinegar, herbs, curry powder
Restricted foods	Meat, fish, eggs, cheese, bread, biscuits, cereal

Table 8.11 continued

Forbidden foods

Puddings	Milk puddings (unless allowed on diet sheet) Ice cream (unless allowed on diet sheet) Ordinary pastry, cakes, sponges (those on Low Protein Recipe Sheet may be taken)
Sweets	Chocolate, toffees, lemon curd, fudge
Beverages	Horlicks, Ovaltine, drinking chocolate, Complan, Bengers, condensed milk, evaporated milk, dried milk
Vegetables	Peas, beans, lentils, sweetcorn
Soup	Tinned, packet or thickened (i.e. lentils, peas, barley, potatoes)
Sauces	Including mayonnaise, salad cream, meat and fish pastes
Nuts	All kinds, peanut butter

8.3.9 LOW SALT DIETS

(a) 50 mmol sodium diets

The majority of patients who need sodium restriction can be managed on the traditional no added salt diet which provides approximately 50 mmol of sodium. Foods which contain high concentrations of salt must be avoided, and examples are shown in Table 8.12. They include processed or cured meats, tinned or smoked fish, tinned vegetables and soups, dehydrated and pre-packed meals, and salted biscuits, nuts and crisps. Additional salt must not be used at the table and only a small amount is permitted during cooking. Provided concomitant potassium restriction is unnecessary a salt substitute such as Salora may be used.

Table 8.12 Examples of foods with a high sodium content

Meat	All processed or canned meats such as bacon, ham, tongue, tinned meat, sausages, hamburgers, haggis, pâté, pies and black puddings
Fish	Tinned fish, smoked fish, shellfish, fish pâté
Cheese	All except cream or cottage cheese
Convenience foods	Tinned vegetables, tinned and packet soups, dehydrated and pre-packed meals
Miscellaneous	Oatcakes, salted and savoury biscuits, salted nuts and crisps, Oxo, Bovril, Marmite, tomato juice, bottled sauces and pickles

(b) 20 mmol sodium diets

Very low sodium diets which contain 20 mmol of sodium are much less palatable. No added salt is allowed at the table or during cooking, unsalted butter should be used and milk is restricted to 250 ml. The forbidden list of foods (Table 8.12) is extended to include all breakfast cereals except Shredded Wheat, Puffed Wheat and Sugar Puffs, cakes and other foods containing bicarbonate of soda, condensed and evaporated milk and ice cream, and sweets such as chocolates, sherbet, toffee and Liquorice Allsorts.

A sample menu for a 20 mmol sodium diet is shown in Table 8.13. Flavourings such as bayleaves, chives, curry powder, garlic, lemon juice, mint, mustard and onions improve the taste of savoury dishes. Some vegetables may taste better when cooked in water containing a small amount of sugar or vinegar. Potatoes taste best baked, fried or roasted, and meats are more palatable when grilled, fried or roasted. Low sodium baking powder can be obtained for home baking.

8.3.10 POTASSIUM-RESTRICTED DIETS

Potassium restriction is important for patients with advanced renal failure who are undergoing conservative treatment or haemodialysis.

Table 8.13   Very low salt diet (20 mmol sodium) sample menu

Breakfast	Fruit, fresh or tinned fruit juice
	Unsalted porridge, Shredded Wheat, Puffed
	Wheat or Sugar Puffs
	Salt free bread with unsalted butter
	Marmalade, jam, honey
	Tea or coffee (using milk from daily allowance)
Mid morning	Tea or coffee (using milk from daily allowance)
	or fresh or tinned fruit juice
	One plain biscuit
Lunch	Soup (only if homemade and unsalted)
	Unsalted meat, fish or poultry
	Unsalted vegetables or salad
	Unsalted potato or rice
	Fruit – fresh, tinned or stewed
	and/or jelly
	and/or milk pudding (using milk from daily allowance)
Mid afternoon	As mid morning
Supper	Unsalted meat, fish, poultry or one egg
	Unsalted vegetable or salad
	Unsalted potato or rice
	Fruit – fresh, tinned or stewed
	Salt free bread with unsalted butter
	Jam, jelly or honey
	Tea (using milk from allowance)
Evening	As mid morning

Patients are given a list of foods which contain high potassium concentrations and which should be avoided: examples are given in Table 8.14. Vegetables should not be eaten raw, rather they require cooking to leach out as much potassium as possible. Before cooking potatoes are soaked for five hours, and they are then boiled in a large volume of water. Roast potatoes must be avoided unless they are first boiled, chips are not allowed. Permitted fruits include water melon,

Table 8.14 Potassium restricted diet: high potassium foods to be avoided

Cereals	Wholegrain breakfast cereals e.g. All-Bran, muesli, Weetabix Wholemeal and brown bread Wholegrain crispbreads e.g. Ryvita Oatcakes
Vegetables	Beetroot, beans – baked, butter and haricot, broccoli, brussels sprouts, baked beans, leeks, mushrooms, spinach, sweetcorn, tomatoes, dry and split peas, lentils. Potatoes – chipped, fried or roast
Drinks	Instant coffee, strong tea Natural fruit juices, tomato juice Oxo, Bovril, Marmite Cocoa, drinking chocolate, Bournvita, Horlicks, Ovaltine Most alcoholic drinks – except spirits
Miscellaneous	Treacle, fruit gums, toffee, chocolate, liquorice, nuts, potato crisps, curry powder, fruit cake, gingerbread
Fruits	Many fruits are high in potassium especially dried fruits e.g. prunes, dates and currants, which must be avoided. Avoid grapefruit, oranges, bananas etc.

apples, lemons, pears, and bilberries. Stewed blackberries, gooseberries and plums can be eaten without any juice. Finally patients who are also on a salt-restricted diet must be warned against using salt substitutes.

8.3.11 GLUTEN FREE DIET

Gluten is present in wheat, rye, barley and oats, thus foods containing these cereals should not be eaten. However some patients with gluten enteropathy may be able to tolerate barley and oats which contain relatively small amounts of gluten, but their inclusion should be carefully monitored. A number of gluten free products are available on prescription, which include gluten free flour, bread and biscuits. Patients with gluten enteropathy should be encouraged to join the Coeliac Society which is a valuable source of information and is responsible for the annual compilation of a list of manufactured foods that are gluten free.

Examples of foods that are allowed and foods to be avoided are given in Table 8.15. Patients must be reminded of the need to check the list of ingredients on packaged foods. A sample gluten free menu is illustrated in Table 8.16.

8.3.12 ELIMINATION DIETS

This type of diet is used in a patient with suspected food intolerance, food allergy or Crohn's disease, and is frequently a source of controversy. An elimination diet is illustrated in Table 8.3 and the use and supervision of such a diet is discussed in Section 8.2.1.

8.3.13 EXCLUSION DIETS

The demonstration of food allergy or intolerance may necessitate specific dietary exclusion. Some illustrative examples of exclusion diets are briefly reviewed. The therapeutic use of such diets requires detailed discussion between the patient and the dietitian. Each patient is provided with a list of foods that are permissible and lists of items that should be avoided, and the need to scrutinize the ingredient lists in all convenience and manufactured foods is emphasized.

(a) Wheat free diet

A wheat free diet differs from a gluten free diet in two respects: some gluten free products contain wheat starch and oats and rye are permissible in the wheat free diet. Patients must check individual brands of manufactured foods such as oat cakes, rye bread, custard powder, beef burgers, ice cream, and instant potato powder for possible wheat products. Ordinary bread, biscuits, cakes, pastries, pasta and spaghetti and all wheat-containing breakfast cereals must be avoided. The same applies to all processed foods which contain wheat: examples includes tinned meats, sausages, fish fingers, cheese spreads, tinned and packet soups. Instead patients may use flour made from

Table 8.15 The gluten free diet

Foods allowed

Gluten free bread, cakes and biscuits made with special gluten
free flour, plus gluten free baking powder
Rice Krispies, Cornflakes, Puffed Rice
Custard Powder, cornflour, arrowroot, ground rice, sago,
tapioca, rice
Gluten free pasta e.g. Aproten macaroni
Meat, fish and eggs. Sauces and gravies if thickened with
cornflour or gluten free flour
Tomor margarine
Lentils, split peas, broad beans
Soup if thickened with cornflour or gluten free flour
Salt and freshly milled pepper
Vegetables – fresh, frozen, dried. Plain crisps
Fruit – all kinds including juices and squash. No orange
Jelly, some brands of ice cream
Jams, honey, marmalade. Boiled sweets, plain and milk chocolate
Tea, coffee, cocoa, Bovril, Marmite

Foods to be avoided

White and brown bread, rye bread, crispbreads, oatcakes,
cakes, biscuits, pastry made with ordinary flour
Porridge, Weetabix, All-Bran, Puffed Wheat, Sugar Smacks
Semolina, Farola
Pasta e.g. macaroni, spaghetti
Meat and fish pastes, cheese spreads, sausages, white and
black pudding, haggis, meat pies, bridies, fish coated with
batter or breadcrumbs. Bisto
Yogurt – some brands contain gluten
Barley
Oxo-cubes, tinned and packet soups
Pepper compound. Baking powder
Potato croquettes, flavoured crisps
Fruit pie filling
Pudding and cake mixes
Filled chocolates e.g. Smarties, Mars Bars
Malted milk drinks e.g. Ovaltine, Horlicks

Table 8.16   A sample gluten free menu

Breakfast
    Cereal e.g. Cornflakes
    Egg or bacon as desired
    Gluten free bread with butter and marmalade
    Tea or coffee

Main meal
    Clear soup or homemade soup
    (thickened with cornflour)
    Meat or fish
    (gravy or sauce to be thickened with cornflour
    or gluten free flour)
    Vegetables
    Potato
    Milk pudding e.g. custard with fruit

Main meal
    Meat, fish, cheese or egg
    Gluten free bread with butter and jam
    Fruit or gluten free cake
    Tea or coffee

---

soya, rice, maize, or potato to make biscuits, cakes or bread. Cornflakes, Rice Krispies, and porridge can also be eaten.

(b) Milk free diet

All foods containing milk protein must be avoided. Tinned and packet foods have to be checked for milk solids, casein, whey and sodium caseinate. Cheese, yogurt, cream, ice cream and butter are prohibited. Milk and butter substitutes such as Wysoy and Tomor margarine are useful.

(c) Egg free diet

Eggs and all products containing eggs are excluded. Eggs are ingredients of various foods including beef burgers, rissoles, fishcakes, pies, cakes and meringues as well as Bournvita and Ovaltine. Many manufactured brands of biscuits are egg free.

(d) Additive free diets

Azo dyes are permitted food colours. They include tartrazine (E102) which is orange/yellow, sunset yellow (E110) and new coccine or ponceau 4R (E124) which is red. In addition benzoic acid (E210) and its derivatives are permitted food preservatives, as it occurs naturally in foods including peas and bananas. Sensitivity to benzoic acid occurs in association with azo dye sensitivity in some patients.

To eliminate these additives it is necessary to base the diet on fresh foods, avoiding all but the permitted manufactured foods. Tartrazine is used widely in canned fish, soft drinks, cakes, biscuits and convenience foods, and it may also be found in medicines and coloured toothpaste. Benzoic acid is found in fruit juices, cider, beer, prunes, greengages, plums and many forms of tinned fruit, and along with peas and bananas they should be avoided.

Finally patients who need salicylate free diets should avoid not only proprietary medicines such as Aspirin and Disprin but also many fruits including apples, bananas, oranges, plums, peaches, melons, gooseberries as well as peas, tomatoes and cucumber.

8.3.14 THE KETOGENIC DIET

The ketogenic diet is occasionally used to facilitate the control of childhood myoclonic epilepsy. The patient is initially fasted for 48 hours, and thereafter half the energy requirement is provided in the form of medium chain triglyceride oil. Energy intake from ordinary food must be restricted to prevent the suppression of ketones. For example the recommended energy intake for a six-year-old boy is 1800 kcal (7.6 MJ). Medium chain triglyceride oil should provide 60% of this, approximately 1000 kcal (4.2 MJ): 1 g of medium chain triglyceride provides 8.3 kcal, hence 120 g of medium chain triglyceride oil is needed. The rest of the diet contributes 800 kcal (3.4 MJ) but a proportion of this will be used in beverages such as Marvel to mix with the oil. Introduction of medium chain triglyceride should be gradual, increasing the amount over a period of one week. The daily requirement should be taken in four equal amounts with the main meals, and in this way the side-effects of vomiting and diarrhoea are minimized.

References

Christie, A. B. (1980) *Infectious Diseases: Epidemiology and Clinical Practice*, Churchill Livingstone, Edinburgh.

Lessof, M. H., Wraith, D. G., Merritt, T. G., Merritt, J., and Buisseret, P. D. (1980) Food allergy and intolerance in 100 patients – local and systemic effects. *Quarterly Journal of Medicine*, **49**, 259–71.

Passmore, R. and Eastwood, M. A. (eds) (1986) *Human Nutrition and Dietetics*, Churchill Livingstone, Edinburgh.

Paul, A. A. and Southgate, D. A. T. (eds) (1978) *McCance and Widdowson's The Composition of Foods*, 4th edn, HMSO, London.

Pearson, D. J. (1985). Food allergy, hypersensitivity and intolerance. *Journal of the Royal College of Physicians of London.* **19**, 154–62.

Workman, E., Hunter, J. and Alun Jones, V. (1984) *The Allergy Diet*, Martin Dunitz, London.

9

DRUGS AND NUTRITION

9.1 The influence of drugs on nutritional status

9.1.1 THE CONSTITUENTS OF DRUGS

The prescription of drugs leads to the ingestion of additional substances which are present in all proprietary preparations as diluents, carriers, colourings or flavourings. For example many antibiotics and common cough suppressants are made up in solutions which contain much sugar. These should be avoided by diabetics and they contribute to the development of dental caries. Drugs such as Ampicillin, Metamucil and Bisacodyl have a high sodium content, and they should not be given to patients who require sodium restriction such as those with cirrhosis or nephrosis. Similarly Penicillin G and salt substitute contain potassium and should be avoided in renal failure. Artificial colourings including tartrazine are used in some preparations, and they occasionally cause problems in patients with urticaria or hyperactivity.

9.1.2 THE INFLUENCE OF DRUGS ON FOOD INGESTION

(a) Drugs and altered taste sensation

Griseofulvin and Penicillamine have long been known to impair taste, possibly through zinc depletion. Captopril is a more recent addition to this list. Some patients with manic depressive psychosis who require Lithium complain of an unpleasant taste sensation called dysguesia.

(b) Drugs which depress the appetite

The anorectic effect of drugs may be intentional or advantageous. Examples include Fenfluoramine amd Metformin used respectively in the management of obesity and maturity onset diabetes in overweight patients. However drug induced anorexia is usually a disadvantage. This particularly applies to cytotoxic drugs which are used in the treatment of malignant disease. Anorexia may also be a feature with non-steroidal anti-inflammatory analgesics, Digoxin and to a lesser extent bulking agents such as bran and Metamucil.

(c) Drugs which increase the appetite

The use of corticosteroids enhances the appetite in the majority of patients. Whereas this may be an advantage in the malnourished subject with Crohn's disease, it is a disadvantage in the obese asthmatic. Appetite stimulation is frequently an undesirable effect of the sulphonylurea group of oral hypoglycaemic agents. Pheno-thiazide and tricyclic drugs also increase the appetite particularly in patients who were previously depressed.

9.1.3 Drugs and nutrient absorption

Antacids such as aluminium hydroxide bind phosphate, and when taken in large quantities they may lead to hypophosphataemia with malaise, paraesthesia and proximal myopathy. A more common problem is the binding of other drugs particularly Tetracycline and ferrous sulphate. Large amounts of bran will bind calcium and zinc, an important cause of depletion only in underdeveloped countries where diets contain over 100 g of fibre. The impaired absorption of Vitamin B12 by biguanides and of folate by Sulphasalazine is not usually of clinical importance unless other causes of malabsorption of these vitamins are also present.

More general malabsorption can follow drug-induced damage of the liver or pancreas, for example with alcohol abuse, or the intestinal mucosa by anti-neoplastic agents or neomycin. Malabsorption may also complicate the use of drugs which suppress gastric acidity and thereby facilitate small intestinal bacterial over-growth. In addition to suppressing the secretion of gastric acid, H_2 antagonists such as Cimetidine and Ranitidine reduce the absorption of Vitamin B12. The sequestration of bile acids by Cholestyramine leads to steatorrhoea, and also impairs the absorption of Vitamins A, B12, D and K as well as folate, calcium, iron, zinc and many drugs that are administered concomitantly.

9.1.4 DRUGS AND NUTRIENT METABOLISM

The therapeutic effect of some drugs depends on their interference with nutrient metabolism, such as warfarin and Vitamin K and Methotroxate with folate. Most drug nutrient interreactions are epiphenomena which are frequently disadvantageous, some examples of which are discussed below.

(a) Beta blockers

Unselected beta blockers impair glycogen metabolism and can precipitate severe hypoglycaemia in diabetic patients who are receiving insulin or sulphonylurea drugs.

(b) Monoamine oxidase inhibitors

Monoamine oxidase inhibitors such as Phenelzine allow tyramine to enter the bloodstream in sufficient amounts to precipitate a hypertensive crisis. Thus depressed patients who require such treatment must avoid tyramine-rich foods like cheese.

(c) Anticonvulsants

The anticonvulsants Phenytoin and Phenobarbitone have long been known to interfere with the metabolism of Vitamin D and folic acid. Increased metabolism of 1,25 hydroxy Vitamin D can lead to osteomalacia and vitamin supplements may be needed. The reason why these drugs are associated with low serum concentrations of folate is less clear but megaloblastic anaemia does not occur unless there is another reason for folate depletion. Consequently folate replacement is not usually required, and indeed its prescription may be followed by an increased incidence of seizures.

(d) Isoniazid

Isoniazid is widely used in the treatment of tuberculosis and it has occasionally been associated with the development of pellagra. It interferes with pyridoxal phosphate, the metabolically active form of Vitamin B6. This impairs Vitamin B6 dependent enzymes such as kynuroninase, which is involved in the oxidation pathway of tryptophan, one of the products of which is nicotinamide adenine dinucleotide (NAD). There is thus increased reliance on dietary niacin, but Isoniazid also inhibits nicotinamide deamidase, an enzyme involved in the utilization of dietary niacin.

(e) Pyridoxine

Interference with pyridoxine can lead to peripheral neuropathy. In addition to Isoniazid, pyridoxine antagonism may occur with Hydrallazine, Penicillamine and oestrogens.

(f) Alcohol

As discussed in Chapter 7, ethyl alcohol interreacts with thiamin, folate and Vitamin B12. Chlorpropamide and Metronidazole may block the metabolism of alcohol resulting in the accumulation of acetaldehyde.

(g) Glucocorticoids

Glucocorticoids have important metabolic effects. They enhance glucose synthesis by promoting protein breakdown thus inducing a negative nitrogen balance, and they also impair the peripheral utilization of glucose. The consequent hyperglycaemia may be enhanced by mineralocorticoid activity which in addition to the retention of sodium and water results in potassium loss and thus impaired insulin release.

(h) Nitrous oxide

Nitrous oxide abusers may suffer from inactivation of Vitamin B12.

9.1.5 DRUGS AND NUTRIENT EXCRETION

Many drugs influence renal excretion. Thiazides and Frusemide respectively increase and decrease the tubular absorption of calcium. Both diuretics lead to the loss of magnesium and potassium in addition to sodium and water. Laxative abuse while increasing sodium and water excretion in the stool will provoke the renal excretion of potassium because of secondary hyperaldosteronism. Salicylates increase the renal excretion of Vitamin C, the ingestion of large doses of Vitamin C provokes oxaluria, and Penicillamine enhances the excretion of calcium and zinc.

The liver also has an important excretory role and this is achieved by synthesis of insoluble conjugates. Some conjugated products are reabsorbed following bacterial decongugation in the intestinal lumen, so antibiotics facilitate excretion by suppressing bacterial activity. This is the reason for oral contraceptive failure during such treatment.

9.2 The influence of nutrition on drug metabolism

9.2.1 THE EFFECT OF DIET ON DRUGS

Drugs susceptible to low pH like Ampicillin, Erythromycin and Pencillamine are best given half an hour before meals to avoid acid secretion. Gastric irritants such as Indomethacin and Prednisolone should be given with food. Drugs like Propranolol and Metoprolol are better absorbed after meals due to food-related increases in splanchnic blood flow and reduced first pass metabolism. Food-induced reduction in gastric emptying which occurs with fatty meals will increase the absorption of drugs which are weak bases such as Amitriptyline and Diazepam. These are better absorbed in the less acidic intestine. Delayed gastric emptying will also increase the metabolism of drugs such as Digoxin, L-Dopa and the penicillins in the stomach with an associated reduction in absorption.

Drugs such as L-Dopa and Methyl Dopa have structures like amino acids with which they share intestinal transport mechanisms. Meals rich in protein will lead to competition for transport between the drug and amino acids and a consequent reduction in drug uptake. A reduction in dietary protein leads to a fall in the renal plasma flow and a reduced clearance of drugs such as Theophyllin. High carbohydrate diets appear to increase drug metabolism. Drug metabolism is also increased by indole compounds which occur in vegetables of the brassica genus such as cabbage and brussel sprouts. Finally patients who consume large amounts of Vitamin E will potentiate the action of Warfarin by depressing coagulation factor synthesis. These observations are interesting but in isolation they are of doubtful clinical importance.

9.2.2 THE EFFECT OF MALNUTRITION ON DRUG METABOLISM

Until recently this subject received little attention. Many of the changes that are known to occur in malnourished patients may be expected to influence drug metabolism. These include changes in the rate and extent of intestinal absorption, alteration in body composition with a proportionate increase in total body water, reduced concentration of albumin and other binding proteins and alteration in organ function with particular reference to the liver, heart and kidneys. Fatty infiltration of the liver may reflect the reduced synthesis of apolipoproteins, and micronutrient deficiencies impair enzyme activity. There is a reduction in cardiac output and renal blood flow and an increased circulation time. Endocrine factors include reduced insulin secretion and thyroid function and increased cortisol concentrations with reduced cortisol binding. Clearly it is difficult to predict how these various factors may influence individual drug handling. Furthermore many malnourished patients are stressed by trauma, sepsis or underlying disease all of which may also affect metabolism.

Studies of antipyrine half life suggest that it is prolonged in patients with protein energy malnutrition characterized by weight loss and hypoalbuminaemia in whom it is corrected by refeeding. Conversely normal antipyrine values are found in patients with energy malnutrition alone, weight loss but normal blood proteins. Patients with protein energy malnutrition have increased rates of elimination of Tetracycline, Phenylbutazone and sulphonamides which have been attributed to reduced drug binding. The pharmacokinetics of Gentimicin appear unaltered in such subjects.

9.3 Drug delivery during artificial nutrition

9.3.1 ENTERAL NUTRITION

Tablets, whole or crushed, cannot be delivered through fine bore naso-gastric tubes, so it is necessary to prescribe all non-parenteral medication in liquid form. This frequently necessitates the interruption of enteral feeding to inject the drug suspensions down the naso-gastric tubes which should subsequently be flushed before feeding recommences. This process is demanding on nursing time and consequently some investigators have studied the compatibility of drugs with enteral feeds. For example it has been shown that Ensure is compatible with Bactrim suspension, Lanoxin elixir, Keflex suspension and Lomotil liquid, but not with Melleril oral solution. Nevertheless, until more is known about drug stability and delivery from such mixtures it is necessary to administer drugs separately from the nutrient solutions.

9.3.2 PARENTERAL NUTRITION

Patients who require parenteral nutrition should not receive parenteral drugs through the central venous catheter which must be reserved solely for the delivery of nutrient solutions. Interruption of the nutrient infusion for intermittent drug administration will significantly increase the risk of catheter sepsis. Because of this problem, the compatibility of some drugs with various nutrient solutions has been studied with a view to adding the drug during the compounding of the nutrient bags in the pharmacy. Heparin and insulin have been delivered in this way for a long time. More recently the addition of Vancomycin for the control of catheter sepsis has been evaluated. However with the exception of insulin the use of the nutrient bag as a vehicle for drug delivery cannot be recommended. Not only is there uncertainty about compatibility and interreactions between drugs and nutrients, but cyclical nutrient delivery poses a significant problem for drug administration.

When parenteral drugs are required they are best administered through a cannula sited in a peripheral vein. Unfortunately some patients who need parenteral feeding have very poor venous access. Under these circumstances consideration should be given to the use of a dual lumen central catheter. One lumen is used exclusively for nutrient delivery, and the second lumen is available for other purposes including drug administration.

References

Altman, E. and Cutie, A. J. (1984) Compatibility of enteral products with commonly employed drug additives. *Nutr. Supp. Serv.*, **4**, 8–17.

Belinger, W. G., Park, G. D., and Sector, R. (1985) The effect of dietary protein on the clearance of allopurinol and oxypurinol. *New England Journal of Medicine*, **313**, 771–6.

Krishnaswamy, K. (1978) Drug metabolism and pharmacokinetics in malnutrition. *Clinical Pharmacokinetics*, **3**, 216–40.

Roe, D. A. and Campbell, T. C. (eds) (1984) *Drugs and Nutrients: The Interactive Effects*, Marcel Dekker, New York.

Shastri, R. A. and Krishnaswamy, K. (1979) Metabolism of sulphadiazine in malnutrition. *British Journal of Clinical Pharmacology*, **7**, 69–73.

Tranvouez, J. L., Lerebours, E., Chretien, P., Fouin-Fortune, I. H., and Colin, R. (1985) Hepatic antipyrine metabolism in malnourished patients: influence of the type of malnutrition and course after nutritional rehabilitation. *American Journal of Clinical Nutrition*, **41**, 1257–64.

INDEX